T0297429

Prostatitis and Its Management

Tommaso Cai • Truls E. Bjerklund Johansen
Editors

Prostatitis and Its Management

Concepts and Recommendations
for Clinical Practice

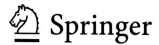 Springer

Editors
Tommaso Cai
Department of Urology
Santa Chiara Regional Hospital
Trento
Italy

Truls E. Bjerklund Johansen
Department of Urology
Oslo University Hospital
Oslo
Norway

ISBN 978-3-319-25173-8   ISBN 978-3-319-25175-2   (eBook)
DOI 10.1007/978-3-319-25175-2

Library of Congress Control Number: 2015957687

Springer Cham Heidelberg New York Dordrecht London

Printed on acid-free paper

Springer International Publishing AG Switzerland is part of Springer Science+Business Media (www.springer.com)

Foreword

After many years of daily involvement in clinical management of urologic patients, I can surely say that prostatitis is one of the biggest clinical challenges within our discipline. The two main characteristics of the disease are its high frequency while – at the same time – limited knowledge is available to the practitioner about the disease and, secondly, its low prognostic severity yet strong impact on their patients' quality of life. This is due to the fact that this urological topic still remains poorly understood, inadequately treated and under-researched. Surely much has changed over the last decades. The initial classification system that was based upon the "4-glass test" has been replaced by a more recent classification system introduced by the National Institute of Health (NIH) focusing on clinical symptoms rather than aetiology which still remains largely unknown. For a long time a validated symptom score was not available, and well-conducted clinical trials were completely lacking. Outcome research has improved our understanding of the incidence, quality of life and economic impact of the disease. Finally, we now have a validated symptom score that appears to adequately measure both symptom severity and response to therapy, and numerous randomized placebo-controlled trials using symptoms as an outcome parameter have been conducted over time which has increased our knowledge on how to improve our management of prostatitis patients. The purpose of this book is to review the state of the art in prostatitis combining practical clinical recommendations with cutting-edge clinical research, basic science and questions for the future. The authors are very well-known experts in the field and have surely based their personal contribution on the most updated scientific evidence without forgetting to share the tricks derived from their precious and vast clinical expertise. Chapters cover the epidemiology and classification of the disease, the diagnostic approach – including imaging studies – and the therapeutic approach to different subtypes of prostatitis. Special focus is reserved for the role of phytotherapy, the management of infective complications following prostate biopsy, the contribution of prostate infection and inflammation to BPH and cancer, the role of STD pathogens in bacterial prostatitis patients and the implications of prostatitis on sexual and reproductive function. It is my sincere hope that the readers will find within this text practical, yet novel, approaches to assist their patients in their clinical practice and come to rely on and refer to it often as a handy reference which enables them to fully recognize, comprehend, diagnose and treat this all-too-common prostate-related pathology.

Vincenzo Mirone
Department of Urology
University of Naples
Naples, Italy

Contents

Introduction and Aim of the Book

1

Tommaso Cai and Truls E. Bjerklund Johansen

Prostatitis is one of the most common illnesses in young men with different clinical presentation such as pelvic pain, lower urinary tract symptoms, or sexual dysfunction and a high impact on their quality of life. The management of prostatitis patients is still today a challenge for the urologist, andrologist, and the general practitioner. The recent acquisitions in terms of epidemiological data and the latest classification from the National Institutes of Health (NIH) have triggered a better management of the prostatitis patient. However, there are holes in our knowledge about the pathophysiology, pathogenesis, and causative pathogens which can make it difficult to find the best treatment for our patients. The need for an improved knowledge is demonstrated by the high number of patients who drop out from scheduled treatments and are lost to follow-up. At the same time, we see a high number of new drugs and phythotherapeutic compounds being introduced in the pharmacopeia and on the market. The situation calls for a standardization of the management of prostatitis patients. On this background, the idea was born to bring together experts in the field to give an update on current knowledge and share practical advices on the management of prostatitis patients. This book aims to provide a comprehensive description of prostatitis, from diagnosis till therapy. This book will be the first handbook addressing all clinical aspects of the prostatitis syndrome and providing the reader with all necessary information to design a tailored therapy. Furthermore, the editors aim to analyze and discuss all relevant clinical implications of the disease, in particular andrological complications (infertility), the possible link between prostatitis and prostate cancer, and infectious complications of prostate biopsies.

T. Cai (✉)
Department of Urology, Santa Chiara Regional Hospital, Trento, Italy
e-mail: ktommy@libero.it

T.E. Bjerklund Johansen
Department of Urology, Oslo University Hospital, Oslo, Norway

Insitute of Clinical Medicine, University of Aarhus, Aarhus, Denmark
e-mail: tebj@medisin.uio.no

© Springer International Publishing Switzerland 2016
T. Cai, T.E. Bjerklund Johansen (eds.), *Prostatitis and Its Management: Concepts and Recommendations for Clinical Practice*, DOI 10.1007/978-3-319-25175-2_1

The final section (questions and answers) is a practical manual for quick consultation in everyday clinical practice. We pay special attention to contemporary aspects of prostatitis related to antibiotic stewardship and elevated PSA: "thoughtless treatment of prostatitis is malpractice, sometimes even a forensic issue." We believe this book will be the first true practical guide for physicians who are involved in diagnostic work-up and treatment of patients suspected of having the prostatitis syndrome. However, it will also serve as a convenient consultancy guide for all physicians who occasionally see prostatitis patients.

Epidemiology and Microbiological Considerations: What's New?

2

Sandra Mazzoli, Tommaso Cai, Marco Puglisi, and Riccardo Bartoletti

2.1   Introduction

Human prostate pathologies are one of the most prevalent clinical conditions with a high impact on social, health-related, and individual costs [1]. In particular, the inflammatory pathologies of the prostate are strongly increasing in males between 20 and 40 years old, with important impact on patient's quality of life [2]. In men of all ages and racial origins, prostatitis prevalence has been estimated to be 10–14 % [3, 4], but there are many biases in the epidemiological studies on prostatitis patients due to several reasons: the lack of a standardized diagnostic tool, the heterogeneity of the clinical presentation, the heterogeneity of the etiology, and the lack of comprehension of the pathophysiology. However, the latest classification of the prostatitis syndromes (National Institutes of Health classification) allows a better definition of the diseases, without a complete resolution of the problem [5].

S. Mazzoli (✉)
Department of Microbiology, Sexually Transmitted Disease Center,
Santa Maria Annunziata Hospital, Florence, Italy
e-mail: mazzoli49@yahoo.com

T. Cai
Department of Urology, Santa Chiara Regional Hospital, Trento, Italy
e-mail: ktommy@libero.it

M. Puglisi
Department of Urology, King's College, London, UK
e-mail: marco.puglisi@apss.tn.it

R. Bartoletti
Department of Urology, University of Florence, Florence, Italy
e-mail: riccardo.bartoletti@unifi.it

© Springer International Publishing Switzerland 2016
T. Cai, T.E. Bjerklund Johansen (eds.), *Prostatitis and Its Management: Concepts and Recommendations for Clinical Practice*, DOI 10.1007/978-3-319-25175-2_2

2.1.1 Epidemiology: International Data

International reports have shown a high heterogeneity that reflects the difficulties in the assessment of the epidemiological data. Roberts et al. estimated that 11 % of Europeans had symptomatic prostatitis [6], while Nickel et al. identified prostatitis in 2.7 % of urological outpatients in Canada with an average age of 50 years [7].

2.1.1.1 European Countries

In Italy, Rizzo et al. performed a national multicenter prospective study on 8503 patients and found a prevalence of prostatitis of 12.8 % (mean age 47.1 years) [4]. Six years later, Bartoletti et al. performed an epidemiological case-control study on prostatitis categories II and III and evaluated the prevalence and estimated the incidence and risk factors of chronic prostatitis/chronic pelvic pain syndrome (CP/CPPS) in urological outpatients in Italian hospitals [3]. From January to June 2006, they enrolled patients from 28 Italian urological centers aged between 25 and 50 years with symptoms of CP/CPPS [3]. Out of 5540 male urological outpatients, 764 were enrolled with CP/CPPS, including 225 (29.4 %) first-visit patients and 539 (70.6 %) who had undergone previous treatment. It was concluded that the prevalence of the syndrome was 13.8 %, while the estimated incidence was 4.5 % [3].

The same results have been reported by Mehik et al. who found a 14 % lifetime prevalence in a cross-sectional Finnish study, in which 27 % of Finnish men reported symptoms at least once per year and 16 % complained of persistent prostatitis symptoms [8].

Finally, in 2007, Marszalek et al. evaluated the prevalence of symptoms suggestive of chronic pelvic pain syndrome in an urban population (Department of Preventive Health of the City of Vienna) and showed that the prevalence of symptoms suggestive of chronic pelvic pain syndrome was 2.7 % without any particular age dependence [9].

2.1.1.2 USA and North American Countries

Statistical data from the National Kidney and Urologic Disease Advisory Board and the National Center for Health Statistics showed that in the USA, prostatitis was ranked fourth among the 20 principal diagnoses made by physicians on referring patients to urologists, and 25 % of urological outpatient visits were due to chronic prostatitis symptoms [10]. Moreover, of almost 32,000 male health professionals in the USA without prostate cancer, 16 % self-reported a history of prostatitis [11]. Notably, during 1 year prostatitis was diagnosed in 12 million men older than 18 years in the USA, including visits made to general practitioners [12]. Among urological outpatients in Canada with an average age of 50 years, 2.7 % were identified with prostatitis, as demonstrated by Nickel [7]. Moreover, Curtis Nickel in a cohort of 868 patients, enrolled in a survey in Canada and analyzed by self-administration of the National Institutes of Health (NIH) Chronic Prostatitis Symptom Index, showed a prevalence of prostatitis-like symptoms of 11.5 % in men younger than 50 years and 8.5 % in men 50 years or older [13].

2.1.1.3 Asian Countries

Tan et al. in 2002 evaluated the prevalence of prostatitis-like symptoms in Singapore, by using a population-based study. They found that the prevalence of prostatitis-like symptoms in a largely Chinese population was 2.67 % [14].

Moreover, in 2013 Wu et al. showed that the prevalence of asymptomatic prostatitis (NIH-IV class) was 21.1 % among 1868 men aged 19–78 years, highlighting that the prevalence of NIH-IV class prostatitis should be taken into account when estimating the total prevalence of prostatitis in future studies [15]. In a cohort of Japanese patients, Kunishima showed that the prevalence of prostatitis-like symptoms was 4.9 % in randomly selected men [16].

Estimated prevalence of prostatitis-like symptoms

Continent	Country	Prevalence	References
Europe	Austria	2.7	[9]
	Italy	12.8–13.8	[3, 4]
	Finland	14	[8]
America	USA	16	[11]
	Canada	2.7	[7]
	Canada	8.5–11.5	[13]
Asia	China	2.6	[14]
	Japan	4.9	[16]

2.1.2 Microbiology: Bacteria and Causative Pathogens

International data showed that only 5–10 % of prostatitis patients have a microbiologically demonstrated bacterial infection [17]. A correct microbiological analysis should include the use of adequate biological material that has to be homogeneous, quantitatively sufficient, and representative of the site infection organ [18, 19]. Collection and sampling have to be simple, noninvasive, and not bothersome for patients, have a good compliance, and have to be not contaminated by a saprophytic microflora. A correct microbiological analysis should also include identification of a low number of bacteria in expressed prostatic secretion or post-massage urines, as this can be the causative agent in chronic bacterial prostatitis [20]. Critical points of microbiological sampling are immediate/rapid transport to suitable conditions for biological materials, immediate/rapid culture after collection, and the application of bacteriological techniques able to quantify a small number of pathogens [21].

The most common isolated pathogens from prostatitis patients are those involved in urinary tract infections (uropathogens), which include: Gram-negative organisms, most commonly *Escherichia coli*, *Proteus* spp., *Klebsiella* spp. and *Pseudomonas* spp., enterococci, *Staphylococcus aureus*, and rarely anaerobic organisms such as *Bacteroides* spp. [17] (Fig. 2.1).

Fig. 2.1 Bacteria involved in prostatitis [17]

Pathogen
Escherichia coli
Other Enterobacteriaceae
Klebsiella spp.
Enterobacter spp.
Proteus spp.
Serratia spp.
Pseudomonas aeruginosa
Enterococci
Enterococcus faecalis
Staphylococci
Staphylococcus epidermidis
Staphylococcus haemolyticus
Corynebacterium spp
Corynebacterium minutissimum
Corynebacterium group ANF
Corynebacterium scminale
Anaerobic bacteria
Lirogenital Mycoplasmata
Ureaplasma urealyticum
Mycoplasma hominis
Other bacteria
Chlamydia trachomatis
Yeasts
Candida albicans
Candida spp.
Saccaromices spp.
Trichomonas vaginalis.

In a retrospective study Mazzoli S. evaluated 1,686 isolated strains from chronic prostatitis patients [17]. The microbiological findings were as follows: 371 strains of Gram-negatives (22.00 %) and 1,112 Gram-positives (65.9 %), 14 yeast strains (0.83 %), and 189 mycoplasmata (11.2 %) [17]. It is worth considering that Gram-positives represented the majority of isolates with strain *Enterococcus faecalis* being the most common with a prevalence of 42.7 % [17]. Similar results have been confirmed by Cai et al. who enrolled more than 15,000 consecutive outpatients with chronic bacterial prostatitis attending a single sexually transmitted disease center from January 1997 and December 2008 [22]. All patients underwent microbiological cultures of first-void early morning urine, midstream urine, expressed prostatic secretion, and post-prostate massage urine. The prevalence of different bacterial strains was stratified in four different periods: 1997–1999, 2000–2002, 2003–2005, and 2006–2008 [22]. In this large cohort of patients, it demonstrated an increasing prevalence of *E. faecalis* strains reaching a peak in the 2006–2008 period [20], highlighting the emerging role of Gram-positive strains [22]. These microbial data follows the widespread use of large-spectrum antibiotics in outpatients.

On the other hand, some cases of prostatitis are caused by atypical pathogens, such as *Chlamydia trachomatis* or mycoplasmata [23, 24]. In fact, a large prospective study of men with chronic prostatitis found that 74 % had an infectious etiology: the most common isolates were *Chlamydia trachomatis* (37 % of cases) and *Trichomonas vaginalis* (11 %), whereas 5 % of patients had infection due to *Ureaplasma urealyticum* [25]. Classical bacterial uropathogens were found in 20 % of patients, and more patients with these pathogens had prostatic specimens with leukocytes as compared with patients with nonbacterial pathogens [25]. Other reports showed that possible prostatitis pathogens include: *Mycoplasma genitalium*, *Neisseria gonorrhoeae*, *Mycobacterium tuberculosis*, various fungi, and several viruses [23, 24]. However, future microbiological studies should be performed in order to clarify the role of atypical bacteria.

2.1.3 The Role of Bacterial Biofilms

The role of biofilm-producing bacteria in the development of urinary tract infections and in acute and chronic prostatitis particularly has been elucidated in recent studies [26, 27]. Bacteria living in a biofilm usually have significantly different properties compared with free-floating bacteria (planktonic) of the same species, as the dense and protected environment of the biofilm allows them to interact in various ways [28]. In this environment bacteria exhibit an increased resistance to antibiotics, as the dense extracellular matrix and the outer layer of cells protect the interior of the community [28]. This aspect is particularly important for the management of chronic bacterial prostatitis patients. Recently, Bartoletti et al. evaluated the role of biofilm-producing bacteria in the clinical response to antibiotic therapy among patients affected by chronic bacterial prostatitis, showing that biofilm-producing bacteria were commonly found and had a significant negative impact on the clinical response to antibiotic therapy [27]. As also highlighted by Tenke et al., this aspect has an important impact on the diagnostic approach. In fact, the diagnosis of chronic bacterial prostatitis can be difficult because colonized bacteria in biofilms will not enter the prostatic secretion or urine sample [29].

In 2006, Kanamaru demonstrated in an "in vitro study" a clear association between acute bacterial prostatitis and biofilm formation [30]. It has been suggested that if bacteria persist after an acute or, more likely, clinically subacute prostate inflammation, they can form small, sporadic bacterial microcolonies or biofilms within the ductal system adherent to the epithelium [31]. There is a quiescent period, a sort of "hibernation," when the environment becomes adverse to and difficult for bacterial existence. The presence of focal sites of bacterial persistence can be postulated by areas of inflammation with subsequent lymphocyte invasion and infiltration of plasma cells and macrophages, which has been demonstrated in both nonbacterial and bacterial prostatitis [32, 33]. It appears that the persistence of bacteria in the prostate gland in these focal biofilms leads to persistent immunologic stimulation and subsequent chronic inflammation. It is suspected that the creation of a chemically and immunologically distinct microenvironment may induce microorganisms to crystallize, calcify, and form calculi [28, 31]. Recently, Mazzoli aimed to isolate potential biofilm-producing bacteria from chronic bacterial prostatitis patients and to evaluate their ability to produce in vitro biofilms [28]. The author evaluated 150 bacterial strains isolated from chronic prostatitis NIH-II patients: 50 *Enterococcus faecalis*, 50 *Staphylococcus* spp., 30 *Escherichia coli*, and 20 Gram-negative miscellanea. Quantitative assay of biofilm production and adhesion was performed according to the classic Christensen microwell assay. Isolates were classified as nonproducers or weak, moderate, or strong producers. The majority of *E. coli*, Gram-negative bacteria, staphylococci, and enterococci strains were strong or medium producers: 63–30 %, 75–15 %, 46–36 %, and 58–14 %, respectively. In this sense, the author highlighted the association between bacteria that were strong producers of biofilm and chronic prostatitis [28]. In line with these "in vitro" observations, Sfanosa et al. demonstrated that acute inflammatory proteins constitute the organic matrix of prostatic corpora amylacea and calculi in men with prostate cancer and presented a definitive analysis of the protein composition of prostatic corpora amylacea and calculi. Moreover, they suggested that acute inflammation has a role in calculi biogenesis: in fact, proteins identified in calcifications, including calprotectin, myeloperoxidase, and a-defensins, are contained in neutrophilic granules [34]. Immunohistochemistry suggested the source of lactoferrin to be prostate-infiltrating neutrophils as well as inflamed prostate epithelium and suggested prostate-infiltrating neutrophils as a major source of protein for calprotectin, because this protein was absent from other prostate compartments. These data confirm the inflammatory genesis and components of prostatic calcifications: inflammation, which resembles the "primum movens" of the calcifications, may now also be the starting point for an additional cascade, amplifying and perpetuating the inflammation itself and the tissue damage. Inflammatory cytokines, especially interleukin 8, were also proved to be present in men with prostatitis as a surrogate marker of prostatitis in general as well as in well-specified *Chlamydia trachomatis* prostatitis [35, 36].

In conclusion and in line with Krieger, most of the published studies about the epidemiological characteristics of prostatitis had important limitations that should be taken into account [37]:

• Few studies include adequate microbiological evaluation.
• Most studies do not include chart reviews or physical examination to assure that subjects do not have the exclusion criteria for chronic prostatitis.
• Most studies rely exclusively on symptom questionnaires or portions of validated symptom assessment instruments. Such surveys are easy to administer, but they are not designed for diagnosis.
• Other urological conditions may present with symptoms that overlap the symptoms of prostatitis.

References

1. Haas GP, Delongchamps N, Brawley OW, Wang CJ, de la Roza CG (2008) The worldwide epidemiology of prostate cancer: perspectives from autopsy studies. J Urol 15:3866–3871
2. Turner J, Ciol M, Von Korff M, Rothman I, Berger R (2004) Healthcare use and costs of primary and secondary care patients with prostatitis. Urology 63:1031–1035
3. Bartoletti R, Cai T, Mondaini N, Dinelli N, Pinzi N, Pavone C, Gontero P, Gavazzi A, Giubilei G, Prezioso D, Mazzoli S, Boddi V, Naber KG, Italian Prostatitis Study Group (2007) Prevalence, incidence estimation, risk factors and characterization of chronic prostatitis/chronic pelvic pain syndrome in urological hospital outpatients in Italy: results of a multicenter case–control observational study. J Urol 178(6):2411–2415; discussion 2415
4. Rizzo M, Marchetti F, Travaglini F, Trinchieri A, Nickel JC (2003) Prevalence, diagnosis and treatment of prostatitis in Italy: a prospective urology outpatient practice study. BJU Int 92(9):955–959
5. Krieger JN, Nyberg L Jr, Nickel JC (1999) NIH consensus definition and classification of prostatitis. JAMA 282:236–237
6. Roberts RO, Lieber MM, Bostwick DG, Jacobsen SJA (1997) Review of clinical and pathological prostatitis syndromes. Urology 49:809
7. Nickel JC, Teichman JM, Gregoire M, Clark J, Downey J (2005) Prevalence, diagnosis, characterization, and treatment of prostatitis, interstitial cystitis, and epididymitis in outpatient urological practice: the Canadian PIE Study. Urology 66:935
8. Mehik A, Hellstrom P, Lukkarinen O, Sarpola A, Jarvelin MR (2000) Epidemiology of prostatitis in Finnish men: a population-based cross-sectional study. BJU Int 86:443
9. Marszalek M, Wehrberger C, Hochreiter W, Temml C, Madersbacher S (2007) Symptoms suggestive of chronic pelvic pain syndrome in an urban population: prevalence and associations with lower urinary tract symptoms and erectile function. J Urol 177(5):1815–1819
10. National Kidney and Urologic Diseases Advisory Board (1990) Long-range plan window on the 21st century. United States Department of Health and Human Services. NIH publication no. 90–583, Bethesda
11. McNaughton-Collins M, Meigs JB, Barry MJ et al (2002) Prevalence and correlates of prostatitis in the Health Professionals Follow-up Study Cohort. J Urol 167:1363–1366
12. Collins MM, Stafford RS, O'Leary MP, Barry MJ (1998) How common is prostatitis? A national survey of physician visits. J Urol 159(4):1224–1228
13. Nickel JC, Downey J, Hunter D, Clark J (2001) Prevalence of prostatitis-like symptoms in a population based study using the National Institutes of Health chronic prostatitis symptom index. J Urol 165(3):842–845
14. Tan JK, Png DJ, Liew LC, Li MK, Wong ML (2002) Prevalence of prostatitis-like symptoms in Singapore: a population-based study. Singapore Med J 43(4):189–193
15. Wu C, Zhang Z, Lu Z, Liao M, Zhang Y, Xie Y, Guo X, Yu X, Yang X, Gao Y, Tan A, Mo Z (2013) Prevalence of and risk factors for asymptomatic inflammatory (NIH-IV) prostatitis in Chinese men. PLoS One 8(8):e71298
16. Kunishima Y, Mori M, Kitamura H, Satoh H, Tsukamoto T (2006) Prevalence of prostatitis-like symptoms in Japanese men: population-based study in a town in Hokkaido. Int J Urol 13(10):1286–1289
17. Mazzoli S (2007) Conventional bacteriology in prostatitis patients: microbiological bias, problems and epidemiology on 1686 microbial isolates. Arch Ital Urol Androl 79(2):71–75
18. Krieger JN, Ross SO, Riley DE (2002) Chronic prostatitis: epidemiology and role of infection. Urology 60(6 Suppl):8
19. Hua VN, Williams DH, Schaeffer AJ (2005) Role of bacteria in chronic prostatitis/chronic pelvic pain syndrome. Curr Urol Rep 6:300
20. Budia A, Luis Palmero J, Broseta E, Tejadillos S, Benedicto A, Queipo JA, Gobernado M, Fernando Jimenez Cruz J (2006) Value of semen culture in the diagnosis of chronic bacterial prostatitis: a simplified method. Scand J Urol Nephrol 40:326

21. Magri V, Cariani L, Bonamore R, Restelli A, Garlaschi MC, Trinchieri A (2005) Microscopic and microbiological findings for evaluation of chronic prostatitis. Arch Ital Urol Androl 77:135

22. Cai T, Mazzoli S, Meacci F, Boddi V, Mondaini N, Malossini G, Bartoletti R (2011) Epidemiological features and resistance pattern in uropathogens isolated from chronic bacterial prostatitis. J Microbiol 49(3):448–454

23. Wise GJ, Shteynshlyuger A (2008) Atypical infections of the prostate. Curr Prostate Rep 6:86–93

24. Lipsky BA, Byren I, Hoey CT (2010) Treatment of bacterial prostatitis. Clin Infect Dis 50(12):1641–1652

25. Skerk V, Krhen I, Schonwald S et al (2004) The role of unusual pathogens in prostatitis syndrome. Int J Antimicrob Agents 24(Suppl 1):S53–S56

26. Bartoletti R, Cai T (2009) Chronic prostatitis and biofilm. Infez Med 17(1):10–16

27. Bartoletti R, Cai T, Nesi G, Albanese S, Meacci F, Mazzoli S, Naber K (2014) The impact of biofilm-producing bacteria on chronic bacterial prostatitis treatment: results from a longitudinal cohort study. World J Urol 32(3):737–742

28. Mazzoli S (2010) Biofilms in chronic bacterial prostatitis (NIHII) and in prostatic calcifications. FEMS Immunol Med Microbiol 59(3):337–344

29. Tenke P, Köves B, Nagy K, Hultgren SJ, Mendling W, Wullt B, Grabe M, Wagenlehner FM, Cek M, Pickard R, Botto H, Naber KG, Bjerklund Johansen TE (2012) Update on biofilm infections in the urinary tract. World J Urol 30(1):51–57

30. Kanamaru S, Kurazono H, Terai A, Monden K, Kumon H, Mizunoe Y, Ogawa O, Yamamoto S (2006) Increased biofilm formation in Escherichia coli isolated from acute prostatitis. Int J Antimicrob Agents 28(Suppl 1):S21–S25

31. Nickel JC, McLean RJC (1998) Bacterial biofilms in urology. Infect Urol 11:169–175

32. Kim DS, Lee EJ, Cho KS, Yoon SJ, Lee YH, Hong SJ (2009) Preventive effects of oligomerized polyphenol on estradiol induced prostatitis in rats. Yonsei Med J 50:391–398

33. Matsumoto T, Soejima T, Tanaka M, Naito S, Kumazawa J (1992) Cytologic findings of fine needle aspirates in chronic prostatitis. Int Urol Nephrol 24:43–47

34. Sfanosa KS, Wilson BA, De Marzoa AM, Isaacsb WB (2009) Acute inflammatory proteins constitute the organic matrix of prostatic corpora amylacea and calculi in men with prostate cancer. Proc Natl Acad Sci U S A 106:3443–3448

35. Lotti F, Corona G, Mancini M et al (2009) The association between varicocele, premature ejaculation and prostatitis symptoms: possible mechanisms. J Sex Med 6:2878–2887

36. Mazzoli S, Cai T, Rupealta V, Gavazzi A, Castricchi Pagliai R, Mondaini N, Bartoletti R (2007) Interleukin 8 and anti-Chlamydia trachomatis mucosal IgA as urogenital immunologic markers in patients with C. trachomatis prostatic infection. Eur Urol 51:1385–1393

37. Krieger JN, Lee SW, Jeon J, Cheah PY, Liong ML, Riley DE (2008) Epidemiology of prostatitis. Int J Antimicrob Agents 31(Suppl 1):S85–S90

The Diagnostic Approach to Patients with Prostatitis-Like Symptoms: What Do We Have to Do?

3

Andrea Benelli and Florian M.E. Wagenlehner

3.1 Introduction

The prostatitis syndrome is one of the most common diseases in urological practice and is the most common urological diagnosis in men under 50 years of age dropping to third place in men over 50 years [1–3]. It includes an important spectrum of entities which are not always easy to identify and to deal with in everyday clinical experience. Due to its growing prevalence and multifactorial etiology, including pathogenic processes outside the prostate (neurological, psychosomatic factors), a significant change in its classification has developed in the last two decades [4]. Prostatitis syndrome has been classified with a consensus process by the National Institutes of Health (NIH) and National Institute of Diabetes and Digestive and Kidney Disease Workshop on Chronic Prostatitis in 1995 [5]. This classification is nowadays used in clinical practice and research and is based on the presentation of symptoms and the presence of white blood cells and bacteria in the expressed prostatic secretion (EPS) [6]. The prostatitis syndrome is classified as acute (category I) bacterial prostatitis (ABP) and chronic (category II) bacterial prostatitis (CPB), chronic pelvic pain syndrome (CPPS) (category IIIA and B), and asymptomatic prostatitis (category IV). The objective of this chapter is to give a practical overview of the diagnostic process in the patient with prostatitis-like symptoms; we will follow the prostatitis classification trying to analyze the most important diagnostic aspects for every category.

A. Benelli
Department of Urology, University of Genoa, Genoa, Italy

F.M.E. Wagenlehner (✉)
Clinic of Urology, Pediatric Urology and Andrology, Klinik und Poliklinik für Urologie, Kinderurologie und Andrologie, Universitätsklinikum Giessen und Marburg GmbH, Justus-Liebig-Universität Giessen, Giessen, Germany
e-mail: florian.wagenlehner@chiru.med.uni-giessen.de

© Springer International Publishing Switzerland 2016
T. Cai, T.E. Bjerklund Johansen (eds.), *Prostatitis and Its Management: Concepts and Recommendations for Clinical Practice*, DOI 10.1007/978-3-319-25175-2_3

3.2   Acute Bacterial Prostatitis (NIH I)

An acute bacterial prostatitis frequently displays as part of an acute urinary infection which involves the prostate and should be thereby considered as a severe systemic infection [1, 7]. The pathogenesis is mostly spontaneous; in some cases (about 10 %) it is a consequence of a urinary tract manipulation such as cystourethroscopy or transrectal prostate biopsy. In this last case enterobacteria such as *Escherichia coli*, nowadays frequently being fluoroquinolone resistant, were found to be the predominant responsible bacteria [8].

3.2.1   Medical History and Physical Examination

A careful medical history and a physical examination are fundamental. The typical presentation includes fever, intense perineal pain, and irritative and/or obstructive voiding symptoms, not rarely evolving into urinary retention [4]. Accompanying epididymo-orchitis and the presence of a prostate abscess are possible complications. Progression to urosepsis is also possible [4, 9]. The physical examination should include palpation of the abdomen to exclude urinary retention and other causes of abdominal pain, scrotal evaluation searching signs of epididymo-orchitis, and a gentle digital rectal examination without prostate massage which is not recommended due to the risk of bacterial dissemination. On palpation the prostate can be also described as hot, tender, and swollen [1, 4].

3.2.2   Laboratory Analysis

The diagnosis is usually suggested by a microscopic analysis of a midstream urine specimen and confirmed by a mandatory microbiological culture which is the only laboratory examination required [1]. If the clinical signs suggest a systemic or even accompanying bloodstream infection, a blood culture is suggested [1, 10]. Enterobacteria (in primis *Escherichia coli*) followed by enterococci and less frequently *Pseudomonas aeruginosa* are the most common pathogenic agents [11].

3.2.3   Imaging

An evaluation of the residual urine with ultrasound is indicated to exclude urinary retention. In patients that do not respond to initial treatment, a transrectal ultrasound (TRUS) of the prostate or a computed tomography can be useful to rule out prostate abscess [12].

3.3   Chronic Bacterial Prostatitis (NIH II)

It is defined as a chronic prostate infection characterized by a history of recurrent urinary tract infections [5]. Its symptoms cannot be distinguished from those of chronic pelvic pain, and only the laboratory analysis can help the differential diagnosis.

3.3.1   Medical History and Physical Examination

A history of recurrent tract infections with previous response to antibiotics can suggest the diagnosis [13]. Often the same pathogenic agent is described and the patient may be asymptomatic between episodes. The symptom complex includes perineal pain, irritative voiding symptoms, and sexual dysfunction due to the physical (pain) and psychological (erectile dysfunction, loss of libido) discomfort [9, 14]. A focused physical examination is mandatory; it should be focused on palpation of the abdomen and on the digitorectal examination (DRE) of the prostate followed by a prostate massage as part of the localization cultures [4].

3.3.2   Laboratory Analysis

Bacteriological localization cultures are fundamental for the diagnosis of chronic bacterial prostatitis [1]. The gold standard is the 4-glass test according to Meares and Stamey; in this test are sampled first-voided urine, midstream urine, expressed prostatic secretion (EPS), and post-prostate massage urine [15]; however, it is a relatively complex and time-consuming examination not always available in the everyday practice. Nickel et al. with patients enrolled in the NIH Chronic Prostatitis Cohort (NIH-CPC) study showed a good correlation of results of the 4-glass test with the 2-glass test, which is a simpler and reasonably accurate alternative nowadays accepted at least for the initial evaluation of patients with chronic prostatitis symptoms [1, 16]. It includes the sampling of a midstream urine before prostate massage and a first-stream urine after the massage. For the diagnosis the bacterial count in the prostatic secretion and/or in the post-prostatic massage urine should be tenfold greater than in midstream [9]. Semen cultures of the ejaculate are not sufficient for the diagnosis because they have a sensibility of 50 % in identifying bacteriospermia [9, 17]. In chronic bacterial prostatitis the spectrum of pathogenic agents is wider than in ABP; a predominant role is played by *E. coli* and the role of intracellular bacteria is still controversial [10].

3.3.3 Imaging and Instrumental Investigations

TRUS can be used in patients with specific indications like the suspect of an intra-prostatic abscess, but it does not help the differential diagnosis of prostatitis [18]. Urodynamic studies may be considered in patients with lower urinary tract symptoms, in the same way cystoscopy or retrograde urethrography may be considered to rule out bladder outlet obstruction [10].

3.4 Chronic Pelvic Pain Syndrome (NIH IIIA–B)

In this category the symptoms should have been present for at least 3 months within the previous 6 months in absence of uropathogens cultured [10]. The NIH classification describes two subcategories: A or B depending on presence or absence of leukocytes in EPS, urine specimen after prostatic massage, or semen [5]. It is nowadays common opinion that the concept introduced in 2004 by the EAU guidelines on chronic pelvic pain panel is adopted, considering this as a multifactorial disease arising from the combination of different pathologic mechanisms, even external to the prostatic gland [19]. The etiology is in most cases unclear; in the last decade five principal causes have been object of studies: infection, detrusor-sphincter dysfunction, immunological dysfunction, interstitial cystitis, and neuropathic pain [9]. The result of such a complex and multifactorial etiology is patients presenting with widely different clinical phenotypes that require a well-structured and standardized, but at the same time flexible, diagnostic process. For this reason and to improve the CPPS management modeling the diagnosis and the therapeutic approach on the multifactorial nature of CPPS, Shoskes et al. elaborated in 2009 the UPOINT(S) system: a clinical phenotype-based classification system including several domains, urinary, psychosocial, organ specific, infection, neurologic/systemic, tenderness of muscles, and sexual dysfunction [20–22].

3.4.1 Medical History and Physical Examination

No single "gold standard" diagnostic test for CPPS exists in the sense of a biomarker [4, 19]. An accurate medical history regarding previous and current diseases and their treatments (medical and surgical) is fundamental. It should be focused on investigating pain and its characteristics (location, severity, duration, and frequency), lower urinary tract symptoms (irritative and obstructive symptoms), sexual dysfunction, and psychological history investigating the quality of life of the patient [4, 9]. The symptoms have to be validated with the NIH Chronic Prostatitis Symptom Index (NIH-CPSI) which explores the most important aspects of this syndrome: pain, voiding symptoms, and quality of life [5]. It is a reliable tool for initial evaluation and therapeutic monitoring, available and validated in many European languages [5, 23, 24]. The IPSS and the IIEF scores represent also a valuable support for initial condition assessment and for the course of the disease in response to treatment [25, 26]. The collaboration with a psychologist can be suggested for these patients helping to explore and monitoring the psychosomatic aspects [27]. Physical examination should also focus on the lower urinary tract including palpation of the abdomen, external genitalia, and perineum and DRE which is particularly important to explore the pelvic floor conditions and to identify any pain trigger point [4, 9].

3.4.2   Laboratory Analysis

At least a urinalysis is useful to exclude microhematuria [1]. The simpler 2-glass test has nowadays replaced in the clinical practice the most laborious 4-glass test with comparable results [15, 16] and together with the ejaculate test can be used to recognize inflammatory and noninflammatory forms [4]. The current thresholds of the Giessen prostatitis clinic for the diagnosis of CPPS are $10\text{--}20/1{,}000 \times$ WBCs in the EPS and $10/mm^3$ WBCs in the post-prostatic massage urine [9, 28]. PSA measurement is not indicated, and urine cytology may be helpful in patients with irritative symptoms to exclude a carcinoma in situ [4, 9].

3.4.3   Imaging and Instrumental Investigations

TRUS can be used if a prostate cyst or abscess is suspected but should not be routinely performed [10]. Urodynamics should be proposed to patients with lower urinary tract symptoms to rule out bladder neck hypertrophy, bladder outlet obstruction, and detrusor-sphincter dyssynergia. A uroflowmetry and residual urine bladder scan should be used for screening purposes and may suggest more differentiated urodynamic investigations [9, 10]. Cystoscopy is not routinely indicated, but becomes mandatory in case of hematuria [10].

References

1. Wagenlehner F et al (2013) Bacterial prostatitis. World J Urol 31:711–716
2. Collins MM et al (1998) How common is prostatitis? A national survey of physician visits. J Urol 159:1224–1228
3. Nickel JC (1998) Prostatitis: myths and realities. Urology 51:362–366
4. Nickel JC (2003) Classification and diagnosis of prostatitis: a gold standard? Andrologia 35:160–167
5. Krieger JN et al (1999) NIH consensus definition and classification of prostatitis. JAMA 282:236–237
6. Schaeffer AJ (1999) Prostatitis: US perspective. Int J Antimicrob Agents 11(3–4):205–211 (discussion 213–216)
7. Schaeffer AJ (2006) Clinical practice. Chronic prostatitis and the chronic pelvic pain syndrome. N Engl J Med 355(16):1690–1698
8. Wagenlehner F et al (2013) Infective complications after prostate biopsy: outcome of the Global Prevalence of Infections in Urology (GPIU) prostate biopsy study 2010 and 2011, a prospective, multinational, multicenter study. Eur Urol 63(3):521–527

9. Wagenlehner F et al (2009) Prostatitis and male pelvic pain syndrome. Dtsch Arztebl Int 106(11):175–183
10. Grabe M et al (2015) EAU Guidelines on urological infections. European Association of Urology Guidelines 2015, limited Update March 2015; 2–86 online http://uroweb.org/guideline/urological-infections/
11. Schneider H et al (2003) The 2001 Giessen Cohort Study on patients with prostatitis syndrome–an evaluation of inflammatory status and search for microorganisms 10 years after a first analysis. Andrologia 35:258–265
12. Ludwig M (2008) Diagnosis and therapy of acute prostatitis, epididymitis and orchitis. Journal Compilation, Blackwell Publishing Ltd Æ Andrologia 40, 76–80
13. Schaeffer AJ et al (2006) Statement on prostatitis. The assessment and management of male pelvic pain syndrome, including prostatitis. International conference on new developments in prostate cancer and prostate disease. Health publications, Paris, pp 343–75
14. Schaeffer AJ et al (2006) The assessment and management of male pelvic pain syndrome, including prostatitis. In: McConnell J, Abrams P, Denis L et al (eds) Male lower urinary tract dysfunction, evaluation and management. 6th international consultation on new developments in prostate cancer and prostate disease. Health Publications, Paris, pp 341–385
15. Meares EM, Stamey TA (1968) Bacteriologic localization patterns in bacterial prostatitis and urethritis. Invest Urol 5:492–518
16. Nickel JC et al (2006) How does the pre-massage and post-massage 2-glass test compare to the Meares-Stamey 4-glass test in men with chronic prostatitis/chronic pelvic pain syndrome? J Urol 176:119–124
17. Ludwig M et al (2000) Comparison of expressed prostatic secretions with urine after prostatic massage–a means to diagnose chronic prostatitis/inflammatory chronic pelvic pain syndrome. Urology 55:175–177
18. Weidner W, Anderson RU (2008) Evaluation of acute and chronic bacterial prostatitis and diagnostic management of chronic prostatitis/chronic pelvic pain syndrome with special reference to infection/inflammation. Int J Antimicrob Agents 31S:S91–S95
19. Engeler DS et al (2013) The 2013 EAU guidelines on chronic pelvic pain: is management of chronic pelvic pain a habit, a philosophy, or a science? 10 years of development. European Association of Urology. Eur Urol 64:43
20. Shoskes DA et al (2009) Clinical phenotyping of patients with chronic prostatitis/chronic pelvic pain syndrome and correlation with symptom severity. Urology 73:538–542, discussion 542–3
21. Magri V et al (2010) Use of the UPOINT chronic prostatitis/chronic pelvic pain syndrome classification in European patient cohorts: sexual function domain improves correlations. J Urol 184(6):2339–2345
22. Magri V et al (2015) Multimodal therapy for category III chronic prostatitis/chronic pelvic pain syndrome in UPOINTS phenotyped patients. Exp Ther Med 9(3):658–666
23. Hochreiter W et al (2001) National Institutes of Health (NIH) Chronic Prostatitis Symptom Index. The German version. Urologe A 40(1):16–17
24. Wagenlehner FM et al (2013) National Institutes of Health Chronic Prostatitis Symptom Index (NIH-CPSI) symptom evaluation in multinational cohorts of patients with chronic prostatitis/chronic pelvic pain syndrome. Eur Urol 63(5):953–959
25. Badia X et al (1997) Ten-language translation and harmonization of the International Prostate Symptom Score: developing a methodology for multinational clinical trials. Eur Urol 31(2):129–140
26. Rosen RC et al (1997) The international index of erectile function (IIEF): a multidimensional scale for assessment of erectile dysfunction. Urology 49(6):822–830
27. Schneider H et al (2005) Prostate-related pain in patients with chronic prostatitis/chronic pelvic pain syndrome. BJU Int 95(2):238–243
28. Ludwig M et al (2003) Chronic prostatitis/chronic pelvic pain syndrome: seminal markers of inflammation. World J Urol 21(2):82–85

Classification of Prostatitis: What Is the Clinical Usefulness?

4

Riccardo Bartoletti and Tommaso Cai

4.1 Introduction

Prostatitis syndrome classification is mainly based on patient clinical characteristics and laboratory findings such as the presence or absence of bacteria and leukocytes in the expressed prostatic secretions of patients with clinical symptoms although its definition includes different types of disease gathered together in a single classification system. Differentiation of patients and their accurate clinical selection seem to be also indicated due to the extreme heterogeneity of available treatments. Symptoms are commonly "generically reported" and consist in the complaint of pain often distributed in atypical locations but always involving the genitourinary tract or other close anatomical areas such as the perineum, the inner part of the thighs, or the lower part of the abdomen. Pain is the most common of symptoms, but others such as urinary symptoms, erectile dysfunction, or premature ejaculation may also be reported from patients. Unfortunately, many urologists tend to use the term "prostatitis" for all patients that are "difficult to diagnose" or with incomplete symptom relief after symptomatic treatments. Therefore, accurate methods for patient characterization and diagnosis are relevant and of high importance for the evaluation of results after administration of different treatments. The prevalence of prostatitis in men between 18 and 50 years has been extensively investigated. About 10 % of men with previous diagnosis of chronic pelvic pain syndrome have a prostatitis. About 10 % of them have a bacterial prostatitis and 0.5 % of them have a sexually transmitted disease with

R. Bartoletti (✉)
Department of Urology, University of Florence, Florence, Italy
e-mail: riccardo.bartoletti@unifi.it

T. Cai
Department of Urology, Santa Chiara Regional Hospital, Trento, Italy
e-mail: ktommy@libero.it

© Springer International Publishing Switzerland 2016
T. Cai, T.E. Bjerklund Johansen (eds.), *Prostatitis and Its Management: Concepts and Recommendations for Clinical Practice*, DOI 10.1007/978-3-319-25175-2_4

prostatitis-like symptoms [1]. Thus, the prostatitis prevalence as well as the criteria used for the optimization, administration, and evaluation of treatments should be seriously considered before the definition of a specific disease classification. Some authors recently supported the theory that patients with psychological problems often report subjective genitourinary and/or sexual symptoms related to their mental condition. Others supported the theory that genitourinary symptoms may induce psychological problems which in turn might influence the sexual behavior. Thus the question is: "Which came first, the egg or the chicken?" [2].

The National Institutes of Health (NIH) classification makes a clear differentiation between bacterial and nonbacterial prostatitis. As a consequence, microbiological diagnosis with Meares four-glass or simplified two-glass test is mandatory in most of patients to obtain the correct arrangement of the disease and prospectively plan the logical and appropriate medical treatment [3, 4].

4.2   The NIH Classification System

The first classification of prostatitis syndromes was proposed by the US National Institutes of Health, National Institute of Diabetes and Digestive and Kidney Diseases (NIH-NIDDK) in 1995. It was subsequently published in 1998. A consensus meeting of the National Institutes of Health Chronic Prostatitis Collaborative Research Network held in May 2002 confirmed the urological research community's approval of this classification system [5] (Table 4.1).

The NIH classification of prostatitis syndromes includes four different main categories:

1. Acute bacterial prostatitis
2. Chronic bacterial prostatitis
3. Chronic prostatitis/chronic pelvic pain syndrome
   (a) Inflammatory
   (b) Noninflammatory
4. Asymptomatic inflammatory prostatitis

Patients with *acute bacterial prostatitis* usually present as acute symptoms of urinary tract infection and in particular frequency and dysuria. Many of these patients may have fever, pyuria, stranguria, pain in the perineal and pelvic areas, and

Table 4.1 The National Institutes of Health classification of prostatitis

Prostatitis NIH categories	Prostatitis type
Cat I	Acute bacterial prostatitis (ABP)
Cat II	Chronic bacterial prostatitis (CBP)

Cat III
  Cat III a
  Cat III b
	Chronic prostatitis/chronic pelvic pain syndrome (CP/CPPS)
	Inflammatory CP/CPPS
	Noninflammatory CP/CPPS

Cat IV	Asymptomatic chronic prostatitis (ACP)

myalgia. Microbiological investigation of urine and semen often reveals the presence of uropathogenic bacteria such as *Escherichia coli* and *Enterococcus* spp. Ultrasonography may demonstrate increased prostate volume and alternance of hypo/hyperechoic areas into the gland. Digital-rectal examination is often contraindicated as well as transrectal ultrasound evaluation in order to decrease the risk of hematogenous and lymphatic spread of infection [6].

Patients with *chronic bacterial prostatitis* may present with recurrent symptoms of infection due to the same microorganisms as mentioned above or less frequently caused by other gram-negative bacteria. Microbiological investigation (Meares two- or four-glass test) allows determination of the causative pathogen species and prescription of appropriate antibiotic treatments. All potentially sexually transmitted microorganisms such as *Chlamydia trachomatis, Mycoplasma* spp., *Gonococci, Trichomonas vaginalis,* and *HPV/HIV* infections should also be investigated in these patients [6]. It is not totally clear if patients with previously diagnosed irritable bowel syndrome and dysmicrobic intestinal flora may have an increased risk of developing prostatic infections [7]. Distinct *E. coli* genomic characteristics have been described in those bacteria found into the urinary tract environment in comparison with those found in the intestinal environment by different authors [8–10].

Prostate calcifications are often seen on prostate gland transrectal ultrasonography investigation, but significant prostate volume increase is not as frequent as in episodes of acute prostatitis [11].

More than 90 % of patients with prostatitis have *chronic prostatitis/chronic pelvic pain syndrome (CP/CPPS)*. Urogenital pain is the most significant complaint. Microbiological investigations are often negative. Other relevant diseases such as urethritis and urethral strictures, cancer, and functional alterations of micturition should be properly investigated before the definitive diagnosis of prostatitis is made [6]. The following diagnostic criteria for CPPS were approved for NIDDK-sponsored research studies on chronic prostatitis [5]:

4.2.1 Inclusion Criteria

- 18 years or older
- Three months or greater duration of pain or discomfort somewhere in the pelvic area

4.2.2 Exclusion Criteria

- The presence of cancer of the genitourinary tract
- Active urinary stone disease
- Herpes of the genitourinary system, bacteriuria (10^5 colony-forming units per ml) in the midstream urine within the past 3 months
- Antibiotic therapy within the past 3 months, perirectal inflammatory disorders
- Inflammatory bowel disease
- History of pelvic radiation or systemic chemotherapy

- History of intravesical chemotherapy
- Documented gonorrhea, chlamydia, mycoplasma, or trichomonas infection of the urinary tract within the past 3 months
- Clinical epididymitis within the past 3 months
- Urethral stricture of 12 French or smaller
- Neurological disease or disorder affecting the bladder
- Prostate surgery (not including cystoscopy) within past 3 months

Prostate calcifications are also frequently seen among these patients on prostate transrectal ultrasonography [11]. Patients with the inflammatory subtype of chronic prostatitis NIH category III have leukocytes in the expressed prostatic secretions, urine after prostate massage, and/or semen fluid. Leukocytes in human semen are usually counted after a histochemical procedure that identifies the peroxidase enzyme and the subsequent presence of $\geq 1 \times 10^6$ WBC/ml (WHO 2010 definition) [12, 13]. Some authors consider this value too high, whereas others consider the counts below the WHO threshold to be associated with deterioration of semen quality [6]. Most leukocytes are neutrophils highly reactive to the peroxidase reaction [12]. Leukocytospermia may be associated with bacterial infection [12]. This is the reason why all these cases should be adequately investigated with microbiological investigations although the Meares test as gold standard method for diagnosis is not so popular among urologists. Conversely patients without evidence of inflammation in the seminal fluid are always classified as noninflammatory subtype category III prostatitis.

Patients with no clinical signs or symptoms of prostatitis (pain and/or urinary and/or sexual complaints) but the presence of leukocytes in the semen are commonly classified in the *asymptomatic inflammatory prostatitis* group (NIH classification category IV). Many of these patients are diagnosed during clinical evaluations for other genitourinary tract issues such as infertility and diagnostic work-up in patients with suspicion of prostate cancer due to raised prostate-specific antigen levels. Inflammatory asymptomatic prostatitis has also been found in the control group of subjects enrolled in observational studies on prostatitis and other prostate diseases. Positive microbiological semen analyses were also found in a limited number of these subjects [6, 14].

4.3 Effects of the Prostatitis NIH Classification

In conclusion, the prostatitis NIH classification seems to be able to objectively characterize patients according to specific criteria, but it is suboptimal to determine the effects of different types of treatment on patient symptoms. Evaluation of seminal fluid content is often difficult because leukocytes are frequently indistinguishable from immature sperms and some of them can also be easily collected from urethral secretions during the ejaculation process. Therefore, it is mandatory to collect the seminal fluid just after the first voided urine prior to ejaculation to obtain reliable results. The histochemical peroxidase enzyme determination is a reliable discriminating factor in the diagnosis of inflammatory disease. Antimicrobials are effective in the treatment of acute prostatitis and chronic bacterial prostatitis. In all these cases besides the clinical improvement of subjective symptoms, repeated microbiological semen analyses are mandatory to demonstrate the complete and permanent eradication of infection. In patients with inflammatory chronic abacterial prostatitis, some infective microorganisms such as *Chlamydia trachomatis* and *Ureaplasma urealyticum* can be easily found in the semen, but their role in the pathogenesis of the disease is still largely debated. Most investigators state that these are not causative agents in abacterial prostatitis. On the other hand, *Ureaplasma urealyticum* and *Chlamydia trachomatis* have been found in about 10 % and 30 %, respectively, of subjects previously diagnosed with abacterial prostatitis by different authors. Some of these patients indeed respond successfully to the treatment with tetracycline or macrolides. In any case, all patients with chronic abacterial prostatitis, which remains the more frequent type of the disease, are difficult to diagnose, treat, and monitor. We need more accurate investigational criteria preferably based on specific symptoms.

4.4   The NIH-Chronic Prostatitis Symptom Index (NIH-CPSI)

The NIH clinical classification includes a systematic evaluation of symptoms in patients with prostatitis. The symptom index is commonly obtained by means of a questionnaire which includes three different domains: pain (questions 1–4), urinary symptoms (questions 5 and 6), and quality of life impact (questions 7–9). Moreover, it is meant to provide a valid index of symptom severity and impact on quality of life for men with chronic prostatitis [15] (Table 4.2).

4.5   The UPOINT Classification

Shoskes et al. recently introduced the novel UPOINT classification to improve the characterization of patients with CP/CPPS (NIH category III prostatitis) [16].

Multiple adjunctive factors such as initial urinary tract infection, intraprostatic urinary reflux, cytokines, pelvic floor spasm, generalized neuropathic or neuroendocrine associations, and psychologic traits should be considered in the scientific evaluation of the pathogenesis of prostatitis. Indeed, none of these factors has been shown to be the sole cause of disease, but a combination of these factors is likely contributing to the pathogenesis of CPPS in the majority of cases, thus characterizing one dominant phenotype in each patient [16]. Men with CPPS present with different symptoms and the intensity of symptoms varies from one patient to another. The UPOINT classification allows separating patients into subgroups, according to the predominant symptoms. The aim of this new classification system is to help the physician in a phenotypic characterization of the disease in order to find tailored and appropriate treatments for each subset of patients. Moreover, the categorization allows appropriate investigations in the treatment monitoring of each subgroup of patients [17].

The UPOINT classification has a six-point system as follows:

- U- urinary symptoms
- P- psychological symptoms
- O- organ-specific symptoms (such as the prostate)
- I- infection-related symptoms
- N- neurologic/systemic symptoms
- T- tenderness in the muscles and pelvic floor symptom

Urinary symptoms are the most prevalent symptoms among patients with CP/CPPS and consist of bothersome frequency, urgency, and/or nocturia. Suggested objective measures include a residual urine volume measurement in order to exclude obstructive symptoms unrelated with CP/CPPS. Therapies include the use of alpha blockers, anticholinergics, dietary changes, and neuromodulation therapies.

Table 4.2 The National Institutes of Health Chronic Prostatitis Symptom Index

Name:	Date:	Date of Birth:	Case No:

1. In the last week, have you experienced any pain or discomfort in the following areas?

a. Area between rectum and testicles (perineum)	2-yes 1-no
b. Testicles	2-yes 1-no
c. Tip of the penis (not related to urination)	2-yes 1-no
d. Below your waist, in your bladder or pubic area	2-yes 1-no

2. In the last week, have you experienced:

a. Pain or burning during urination	2-yes 1-no
b. Pain or discomfort during or after sexual climax (ejaculation)	2-yes 1-no

3. How often have you had pain or discomfort in any of these areas over the last week?

a. Never 1

b. Rarely 2

c. Sometimes 3

d. Often 4

e. Usually 5

f. Always 6

4. Which number best describes your AVERAGE pain or discomfort on the days that you had it, over the last week?

1 2 3 4 5 6 7 8 9 10

No Pain	Pain As Bad as You Can Imagine

Table 4.2 (continued)

Urination

5. How often have you had a sensation of not emptying your bladder completely after you finish urinating, over the last week?

a. Not at all	0
b. Less than 1 times in 5.	1
c. Less than half the time.	2
d. About half the time.	3
e. More than half the time.	4
f. Almost always.	5

6. How often have you had to urinate again less than two hours after you finished urinating, over the last week?

a. Not at all	0
b. Less than 1 times in 5.	1
c. Less than half the time.	2
d. About half the time.	3
e. More than half the time.	4
f. Almost always.	5

Impact of Symptoms

7. How much have your symptoms kept you from doing things you would usually do, over the last week?

a. None	0
b. Only a little	1
c. Some	2
d. A lot	3

8. How much did you think about your symptoms, over the last week?

a. None	0
b. Only a little	1
c. Some	2
d. A lot	3

Psychosocial complaints are frequently reported by patients with pain and maladaptive coping mechanisms (such as catastrophizing), depression, anxiety, and stress. In all these cases, the treatment would include counseling, cognitive behavioral therapy, and antidepressant medications.

Organ-specific symptoms are not uncommon in patients with long-standing pain symptoms. Patients with an organ-specific phenotype would be identified with pain localized to the prostate on digital-rectal examination and to the bladder if pain would be increased during the filling and emptying phases.

Infection symptoms are not frequently investigated in the medical history of patients with CP/CPPS. One of the reasons is that empiric antibiotic treatments are frequently overused and ineffective. Other patients with bacterial infection have been often improperly treated with antimicrobials, and the results obtained with the expressed prostate secretion culture may be indicative of persistent infection and may be successfully treated with antibiotics. In other cases, as previously described, atypical infective microorganisms such as *Chlamydia trachomatis* or *Mycoplasma* spp. may be found in the EPS or the urethral secretions by the Meares-Stamey test and successfully treated with proper antibiotic treatments.

Neurological/systemic conditions such as autonomic dysfunctions and peripheral and central nervous system sensitization (neuropathic) may influence CP/CPPS symptoms. These include irritable bowel syndrome, fibromyalgia, vulvodynia, chronic fatigue syndrome, migraine headaches, and low back/leg pain. Patients with neurological/systemic phenotype may be successfully treated by specific therapies for these conditions, some neuroleptic medications and complementary neuromodulation such as acupuncture.

Tenderness of muscles of subjective and clinical evaluation is particularly significant and relevant in patients with CP/CPPS. Abnormal findings such as muscle spasms or fascial trigger points in the muscles of the abdominal wall, perineum, and pelvic floor can be found through an accurate medical examination. Specific therapies include physical activity, stress reduction, and behavior modification.

Zhao et al. recently reported the results obtained in a single clinical cohort of 389 patients with median age 43 years with a median duration of symptoms of 9.3 months. The median number of positive UPOINT domains was 3. The rate of patients with one positive domain was 5.4 %, with 2 domains 31.6 %, with 3 domains 42.9 %, with 4 domains 13.1 %, and with 5 and 6 domains 5.1 and 1.8 %, respectively. No patient had zero positive domains [18]. In another clinical setting, 22 % of patients with CPPS had symptoms limited to a single domain. The rate of patients with symptoms in a single domain ranged from 52 % of patients with urinary symptoms to 16 % of patients experiencing infection-related symptoms [19]. More recently, a seventh domain has been proposed for symptoms related to sexual function [20]. The original six domains of the UPOINT classification can be easily arrayed as a snowflake-like diagram by using a specific software at the website: www.upointmd.com [20]. This website may help urologists to check and monitor patients prior and after treatment according to their specific CPPS phenotype. Current validation studies confirm that the UPOINT classification remains internally consistent with the exception of the organ-specific category, which seems to contain two separate subgroups: one for men predominantly with bladder symptoms and one for those with prostate symptoms. Some recent results indicated that the six UPOINT classical domains interrelate or cluster into two major divisions. Patients with symptoms in any one of the three categories that are specific to the pelvis (urinary, organ specific, tenderness) have more in common. Conversely, men with symptoms that are predominantly in one of the three systemic domains (neurologic, infection related, and psychosocial) seem to have a common bond [19]. Recent data shows excellent clinical results obtained in patients with CPPS and classified according to the UPOINT classification. The response rate was 84 % with a significant decrease of the NIH-CPSI score [19].

Conclusions

Prostatitis syndromes remain difficult-to-diagnose and difficult-to-treat diseases. According to a definition provided by J.N. Krieger, "Prostatitis is the diagnosis given to a large group of men who present with a variety of complaints referable to the lower urogenital tract and perineum." All patients should be accurately investigated with appropriate clinical investigations to obtain useful information for an adequate NIH classification. Antimicrobial treatments have been demonstrated equally efficient in the treatment of cat. I-II diseases as in a few cases of cat.III disease. The UPOINT phenotyping in the case of chronic abacterial prostatitis allows tailoring of appropriate treatments with encouraging results in terms of clinical response and therapeutic success.

References

1. Grabe M, Bartoletti R, Bjerklund-Johansen TE, Cek M, Koves B, Naber KG, Pickard RS, Tenke P, Wagenlehner F, Wullt B (2015) EAU guidelines on urological infections. The European association of Urology, Arnhem (NL). 2015 edn, pp 42–46. http://uroweb.org/wp-content/uploads/19-Urological-infections_LR2.pdf
2. Tripp DA, Nickel JC, Wang Y, Litwin MS, McNaughton-Collins M, Landis JR, Alexander RB, Schaeffer AJ, O'Leary MP, Pontari MA, Fowler JEJ, Nyberg LM, Kusek JW (2006) Catastrophizing and pain-contingent rest predict patient adjustment in men with chronic prostatitis/chronic pelvic pain syndrome. J Pain 7:697
3. Krieger JN, Egan KJ, Ross SO et al (1996) Chronic pelvic pain represent the most prominent urogenital symptoms of "chronic prostatitis". Urology 48:715–722
4. Meares EM, Stamey TA (1968) Bacteriologic localization patterns in bacterial prostatitis and urethritis. Invest Urol 5:492–518
5. Krieger JN, Nyberg L Jr, Nickel CJ (1999) NIH consensus definition and classification of prostatitis. JAMA 281(3):236–237
6. Schaeffer AJ (1999) Prostatitis: US perspective. Int J Antimicrob Agents 11:2015–2211
7. Bullones Rodriguez MA, Afari N, Buchwald DS, the NIDDK diseases working group on Urological Chronic Pelvic Pain (2013) Evidence for overlap between urological and nonurological unexplained clinical conditions. J Urol 189(Suppl 1):S66–S74
8. Welch RA, Burland V, Plunkett III G, Redford P, Roesch P, Rasko D, Buckles EL, Liou SR, e collaboratori (2002) Extensive mosaic structure revealed by the complete genome sequence of uropathogenic E. coli. Proc Natl Acad Sci U S A 99:17020–17024
9. Cottell E, Harrison RF, McCaffrey M, Walsh T, Mallon E, Barry-Kinsella C (2000) Are seminal fluid microorganism of significance or merely contaminants? Fertil Steril 74:465–470
10. Gandaglia G, Briganti A, Gontero P, Mondaini N, Novara G, Salonia A, Sciarra A, Montorsi F (2013) The role of chronic prostatic inflammation in the pathogenesis and progression of benign prostatic hyperplasia (BPH). BJU Int 112:432–441
11. Weidner W, Anderson RU (2008) Evaluation of acute and chronic bacterial prostatitis and diagnostic management of chronic prostatitis/chronic pelvic pain syndrome with special reference to infection/inflammation. Int J Antimicrob Agents (31 Supp 1):S91–5
12. WHO (2010) WHO laboratory manual for the examination and processing of human semen, 5th edn. WHO press, Geneva
13. Bartoletti R, Cai T, Mondaini N, Dinelli N, Pinzi N, Pavone C, Gontero P, Gavazzi A, Giubilei G, Prezioso D, Mazzoli S, Boddi V, Naber KG, Italian Prostatitis Study Group (2007) Prevalence, incidence estimation, risk factors and characterization of chronic prostatitis/chronic pelvic pain syndrome in urological hospital outpatients in Italy: results of a multicenter case-control observational study. J Urol 178(6):2411–2415; discussion 2415
14. Litwin MS, McNaughton-Collins M, Fowler FJ Jr, Nickel JC, Calhoun EA, Pontari MA, Alexander RB, Farrar JT, O'Leary MP (1999) The National Institutes of Health chronic prostatitis symptom index: development and validation of a new measure. Chronic prostatitis collaborative research network. J Urol 162(2):369–375
15. Shoskes DA, Nickel JC, Rackley RR, Pontari MA (2009) Clinical phenotyping in chronic prostatitis/chronic pelvic pain syndrome and interstitial cystitis: a management strategy for urologic chronic pelvic pain syndromes. Prostate Cancer Prostatic Dis 12(2):177–183

16. Shoskes DA, Nickel JC (2013) Classification and treatment of men with chronic prostatitis/chronic pelvic pain syndrome using the UPOINT system. World J Urol 31:755–760
17. Zhao Z, Zhang J, He J, Zeng G (2013) Clinical utility of the UPOINT phenotype system in chinese males with chronic prostatitis/chronic pelvic pain syndrome (CP/CPPS): a prospective study. PLoS One 8:e52044
18. Shoskes DA, Nickel JC, Dolinga R, Prots D (2009) Clinical phenotyping of patients with chronic prostatitis/chronic pelvic pain syndrome and correlation with symptom severity. Urology 73:538–542
19. Magri V, Wagenlehner F, Perletti G, Schneider S, Marras E, Naber KG, Weidner W (2010) Use of the UPOINT chronic prostatitis/chronic pelvic pain syndrome classification in European patient cohorts: sexual function domain improves correlations. J Urol 184:2339–2345
20. Upoint system for the clinical phenotyping of chronic pelvic pain. www.upointmd.com

Imaging Studies: What Is Their Role?

5

N. Pavan, S. Rai, F. Vedovo, M. Bertolotto, M. Iannelli,
C. Trombetta, and G. Liguori

5.1   Introduction

Beyond the use of gray scale and color Doppler modes, other imaging modalities may be indicated for imaging prostatitis in selected cases. Contrast-enhanced ultrasonography (CEUS) has potential in differentiating avascular abscesses from hypovascular lesions and in identifying small abscesses not detected on conventional ultrasonographic modes. Multiparametric MR imaging allows a panoramic view of the prostate and of the surrounding tissues, which may be useful in severe inflammation spreading outside the boundaries of the organ. T2-weighted, diffusion-weighted, and T1-weighted images with fat suppression obtained after intravenous paramagnetic contrast agent injection are of particular value. While signal intensity

N. Pavan (✉)
Urology Clinic, Department of Medical, Surgical and Health Science,
University of Trieste, 447 Strada di Fiume 34149, Trieste, Italy

Department of Urology, University of Miami Miller School of Medicine and Sylvester
Comprehensive Cancer Center, Miami, FL, USA
e-mail: nicpavan@gmail.com

S. Rai
Department of Urology, University of Miami Miller School of Medicine and
Sylvester Comprehensive Cancer Center,
Miami, FL, USA

F. Vedovo • C. Trombetta • G. Liguori
Urology Clinic, Department of Medical, Surgical and Health Science, University of Trieste,
447 Strada di Fiume 34149, Trieste, Italy
e-mail: gioliguori@libero.it

M. Bertolotto • M. Iannelli
Department of Radiology, Surgical and Health Science, University of Trieste,
447 Strada di Fiume 34149, Trieste, Italy

© Springer International Publishing Switzerland 2016
T. Cai, T.E. Bjerklund Johansen (eds.), *Prostatitis and Its Management: Concepts
and Recommendations for Clinical Practice*, DOI 10.1007/978-3-319-25175-2_5

of the peripheral normal prostate is usually high in T2-weighted images, inhomogeneous reduction is observed in prostatitis. Moreover, enhancement of the gland increases, as well as that of surrounding tissues involved by the inflammatory process. Diffusion-weighted images provide information about motion of the water molecules, which is restricted in collections of dense fluid such as pus. Indeed, abscesses usually present with relatively high signal intensity on T2-weighted images, but lower than water, and high signal intensity on diffusion-weighted images. Vascularization is lacking after gadolinium contrast administration. A perilesional rim of enhancement may be observed. Air is signal void in all MR sequences.

5.2   Acute Prostatitis

The measuring of post-void urinary residue should routinely be carried out in the first 24 h, whether by ultrasonography (US) or by using bladder scan. If the amount is significant, urinary drainage via a suprapubic catheter is indicated. True radiological investigations are only indicated where there is suspicion of possible pyelonephritis or in persistent cases or indeed in patients who deteriorate and develop sepsis within 72 h, to investigate possible complications [1].

Some authors recommend that suprapubic pelvic sonography should be carried out in view of the pain that patients present and the risk of bacteremia [2]. In 80 % of cases, this would allow detection of one or several abnormalities: increased prostate size, enlarged venous plexus, and hypoechoic site of inflammation with focal or diffuse increased vascularization visualized on Doppler scanning (Fig. 5.1). However, the real aim of sonography is to check whether there is a prostatic abscess (Fig. 5.2): this is visualized as a nonhomogenous and moderately hypoechoic rounded lesion, with septations and thick walls and with increased vascularization on Doppler scanning, although the center is avascular. It is then also possible to

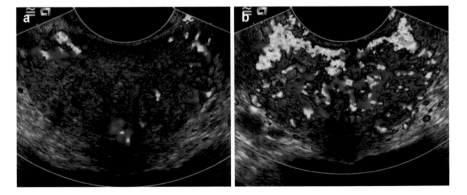

Fig. 5.1 Color Doppler appearance of the prostate gland. Transrectal transverse scans. (**a**) Normal prostate. (**b**) Patient with clinically obvious prostatitis showing marked hypervascularization of the prostate gland

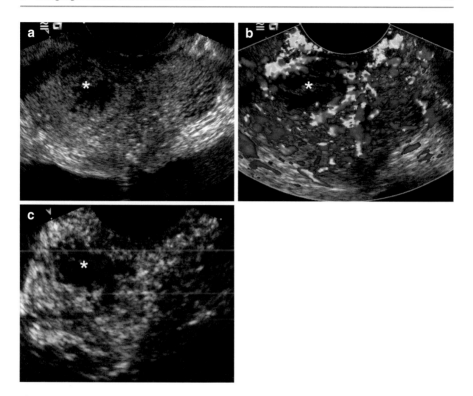

Fig. 5.2 Clinically obvious severe acute prostatitis complicated with abscess formation. Transrectal transverse scans. (**a**) Gray scale ultrasonography shows a lesion with mixed echogenicity (*asterisk*) in the right lobe of the prostate. (**b**) Color Doppler interrogation shows lack of vascularity of the lesion (*asterisk*) and marked hypervascularization of the right prostate lobe. (**c**) CEUS confirms complete lack of vascularization of lesion (*asterisk*) and avid enhancement of the surrounding prostate parenchyma, consistent with abscess formation

drain the abscess under transperineal or transrectal ultrasound guidance. An examination of the whole genitourinary system is indicated in order to check for signs of orchitis, epididymitis, or complicated pyelonephritis [3]. MR should be performed in selected cases to evaluate the extension of the inflammatory process to the surrounding tissues (Figs. 5.3 and 5.4).

5.3 Chronic Prostatitis

Sonography may be normal and reveal totally nonspecific abnormalities: numerous calcifications often accumulate in the posterolateral regions of the peripheral prostate; increased vascularization is not detectable on current sonography equipment; the echostructure of the prostatic parenchyma is nonhomogenous, alternating

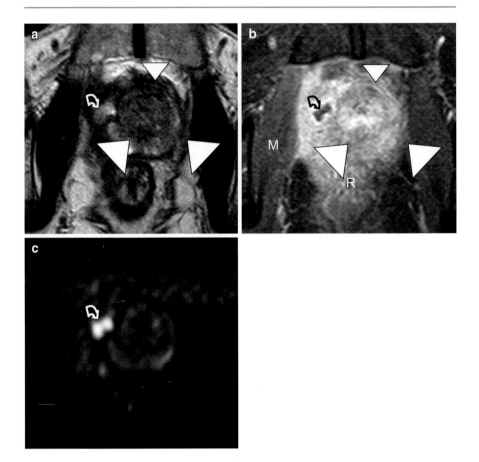

Fig. 5.3 Clinically obvious severe prostatitis investigated with MR imaging performed to evaluate the extension of the inflammatory process to the surrounding tissues. Axial images of the prostate gland. (**a**) T2-weighted image showing inhomogeneously hypointense gland (*arrowheads*). A hyperintense lesion is detected in the right lobe (*curved arrow*). (**b**) T1-weighted image with fat suppression obtained after intravenous gadolinium contrast administration shows avid enhancement of the prostate gland (*arrowheads*) and of the right periprostatic tissues spreading laterally to the obturator internus muscle (*M*) and posteriorly to the rectum (*R*). The lesion in the right lobe (*curved arrow*) displays lack of internal vascularity and perilesional rim of enhancement, consistent with abscess formation. (**c**) Diffusion-weighted image confirms diagnosis of prostatic abscess showing signal restriction (*curved arrow*), consistent with pus

between non-systematized hyperechoic strips and hypoechoic zones that sometimes contain pseudonodules and dilated ducts [4].

Faced with a hypoechoic strip in the peripheral zone, differential diagnosis from an underlying neoplasm is impossible and an ultrasound-guided biopsy is required depending on the context. MRI is not indicated for the positive diagnosis of chronic prostatitis, but when it is used to guide a prostate biopsy in a patient with raised PSA levels or to assess disease spread in a known cancer, it usually allows cancer to be distinguished from chronic prostatitis [5].

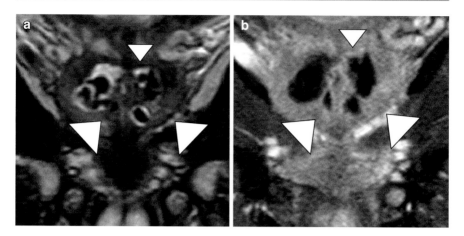

Fig. 5.4 Incidental detection of multiple prostatic abscesses in an AIDS patient presenting with perianal pain and no significant signs of inflammation. MR imaging was performed to rule out perianal fistulas. Coronal images of the prostate gland (*arrowheads*). (**a, b**) T2-weighted (**a**) and T1-weighted image with fat suppression (**b**) obtained after intravenous paramagnetic contrast administration showing multiple air-containing abscess cavities (signal void areas in both images)

5.4   Granulomatous Prostatitis

Granulomatous prostatitis (GP), a benign inflammatory condition of the prostate, is a rare urological disorder [6]. First described by Tanner and McDonald in 1943, it has an incidence of 3.3 % among inflammatory lesions [7]. However, some studies report that a significant percentage of men receiving intravesical Bacillus Calmette-Guérin (BCG) immunotherapy for the treatment of superficial urothelial carcinoma of the bladder develop granulomatous prostatitis [8, 9]. The most commonly reported signs are cystic dilation of the ducts, secondary to stenosis of the ejaculatory ducts, and these can meet with the urethra taking on an appearance of cavitation [10–11]. It is generally combined with macro calcifications [6, 7]. Sonography demonstrates single or multiple hypoechoic nodules, localized to the peripheral zone. Since it has a similar clinical presentation and transrectal ultrasound (TRUS) appearance to that of carcinoma of the prostate (CaP) [12, 13] and is associated with an increase in serum prostate-specific antigen (PSA), BCG-induced GP may be mistaken for CaP [14–18].

Several studies have investigated the role of magnetic resonance imaging (MRI) in order to find any specific features that may help differentiate between GP and CaP, thereby eliminating the need of performing an invasive prostate biopsy to get an accurate diagnosis. GP has been shown to have a generalized tumorlike appearance with hypo-signal intensity on T2WI in peripheral zone foci [19–21], similar to that of CaP. Naik and Carey [16] evaluated the MR images of 10 patients with histologically proven GP diagnosed by TRUS and biopsy and concluded that MRI failed to establish a specific diagnosis of GP or differentiate it from CaP. However, Kawada et al. [22] used multiphase contrast-enhanced MRI to evaluate the features of GP in five patients with histopathologically proven GP and demonstrated an early and prolonged ring enhancement on gadolinium-enhanced MRI, which might be a key finding in helping differentiate GP from CaP.

References

1. Roy C (2005) Imagerie de la prostate. Elsevier Masson, Paris
2. Cornud F (2004) Imagerie de la prostate. Sauramps Médical, Paris
3. Schull A, Monzani Q, Bour L, Barry-Delongchamps N, Beuvon F, Legmann P, Cornud F (2012) Imaging in lower urinary tract infections. Diagn Interv Imaging 93(6):500–508
4. Ludwig M, Weidner W, Schroeder-Printzen I, Zimmermann O, Ringert R (1994) Transrectal prostatic sonography as a useful diagnostic means for patients with chronic prostatitis or prostatodynia. Br J Urol 73(6):664–668
5. Hélénon O, Bellin MF, Claudon M, Collectif CF (2005) Imagerie de l'appareil génito-urinaire: appareil urinaire, appareil génital masculin. Flammarion médecinesciences, Paris
6. Carrero Lopez VM, Rodriguez Antolin A, Caballero J et al (1994) Granulomatous prostatitis. An infrequent diagnosis. Review of our series. Actas Urol Esp 18:77–84
7. Tanner FH, McDonald JR (1943) Granulomatous prostatitis: a histologic study of a group of granulomatous lesions collected from prostate glands. Arch Pathol Lab Med 36:358–370
8. LaFontaine PD, Middleman BR, Graham SD Jr, Sanders WH (1997) Incidence of granulomatous prostatitis and acid-fast bacilli after intravesical BCG therapy. Urology 49:363–366
9. Oates RD, Stilmant MM, Freedlund MC, Siroky MB (1988) Granulomatous prostatitis following bacillus Calmette-Guérin immunotherapy of bladder cancer. J Urol 140:751–754
10. Matos MJ, Bacelar MT, Pinto P, Ramos I (2005) Genitourinary tuberculosis. Eur J Radiol 55(2):181–187
11. Jung YY, Kim JK, Cho K-S (2005) Genitourinary tuberculosis: comprehensive cross-sectional imaging. AJR Am J Roentgenol 184(1):143–150
12. Clements R, Gower Thomas K, Griffiths GJ, Peeling WB (1993) Transrectal ultrasound appearances of granulomatous prostatitis. Clin Radiol 47:174–176
13. Rubenstein JB, Swayne LC, Magidson JG, Furey CA (1991) Granulomatous prostatitis: a hypoechoic lesion of the prostate. Urol Radiol 13:119–122
14. Lamm DL, Stogdill VD, Stogdill BJ, Crispen RG (1986) Complications of bacillus Calmette-Guerin immunotherapy in 1,278 patients with bladder cancer. J Urol 135:272–274
15. Miyashita H, Troncoso P, Babaian RJ (1992) BCG-induced granulomatous prostatitis: a comparative ultrasound and pathologic study. Urology 39:364–367
16. Naik KS, Carey BM (1999) The transrectal ultrasound and MRI appearances of granulomatous prostatitis and its differentiation from carcinoma. Clin Radiol 54:173–175
17. Gevenois PA, Stallenberg B, Sintzoff SA, Salmon I, Van Rogemorter G, Struyven J (1992) Granulomatous prostatitis: a pitfall in MR imaging of prostatic carcinoma. Eur Radiol 2:365–367
18. Takeuchi M, Suzuki T, Sasaki S, Ito M, Hamamoto S, Kawai N et al (2012) Clinicopathologic significance of high signal intensity on diffusion-weighted MR imaging in the ureter, urethra, prostate and bone of patients with bladder cancer. Acad Radiol 19:827–833
19. Suzuki T, Takeuchi M, Naiki T, Kawai N, Kohri K, Hara M et al (2013) MRI findings of granulomatous prostatitis developing after intravesical Bacillus Calmette-Guérin therapy. Clin Radiol 68:595–599
20. Oppenheimer JR, Kahane H, Epstein JI (1997) Granulomatous prostatitis on needle biopsy. Arch Pathol Lab Med 121:724–729
21. Bour L, Schull A, Delongchamps NB, Beuvon F, Muradyan N, Legmann P et al (2013) Multiparametric MRI features of granulomatous prostatitis and tubercular prostate abscess. Diagn Interv Imaging 94:84–90
22. Kawada H, Kanematsu M, Goshima S, Kondo H, Watanabe H, Noda Y, Tanahashi Y, Kawai N, Hoshi H (2015) Multiphase contrast-enhanced magnetic resonance imaging features of Bacillus Calmette-Guérin-induced granulomatous prostatitis in five patients. Korean J Radiol 16(2):342–348

Treatment of Bacterial Prostatitis: Clinico-Pharmacological Considerations

6

Gianpaolo Perletti and Vittorio Magri

6.1 Acute Bacterial Prostatitis

Acute bacterial prostatitis (ABP, Category I, NIH classification [27]) shows high rates of response to therapy and high likelihood of cure and hence is reputed to be an easy-to-manage infection. In fact, contrary to its chronic counterpart, ABP responds well to therapy with broad-spectrum beta-lactam antibiotics like penicillins and cephalosporins. It is believed that the intercellular microenvironment of an acutely infected prostate may become permissive to the diffusion and distribution of a number of drugs. In fact, there is empirical evidence that, similar to the scenario occurring in the case of brain infections, where inflammation partially disrupts the blood-brain barrier, ABP-induced inflammation may alter the tight adhesion of prostate glandular cells, thus allowing various antibacterial agents, including beta-lactams, to "leak" through intercellular spaces, easily reaching the ductal/luminal sites of infection.

Despite prompt responsiveness to antibiotics, ABP is a serious condition, occasionally requiring treatment in an inpatient setting due to the risk of onset of severe complications like life-threatening urosepsis, or to the likelihood of evolving into category II *chronic bacterial prostatitis* (CBP) or category III *chronic prostatitis/ chronic pelvic pain syndrome* (CP/CPPS).

ABP is often caused by ascending urethral colonization, but other spread modalities have been described for this infection, for example, direct seeding from

G. Perletti (✉)
Laboratory of Toxicology and Pharmacology, Biomedical Research Division,
Department of Theoretical and Applied Sciences, Università degli Studi dell'Insubria,
Busto Arsizio, Varese, Italy
e-mail: gianpaolo.perletti@uninsubria.it

V. Magri
Urology Secondary Care Clinic, Azienda Ospedaliera Istituti Clinici di Perfezionamento,
Milan, Italy

© Springer International Publishing Switzerland 2016
T. Cai, T.E. Bjerklund Johansen (eds.), *Prostatitis and Its Management: Concepts and Recommendations for Clinical Practice*, DOI 10.1007/978-3-319-25175-2_6

transrectal prostate biopsy procedures. Factors predisposing to ABP can be unprotected sexual intercourse, urinary catheterization, use of transurethral instrumentation, and other procedures that may facilitate the delivery of pathogens to the prostate gland in an ascending fashion.

ABP presents in most cases with an array of characteristic features, including fever, chills, and malaise, accompanied by specific urinary irritative and/or obstructive symptoms and signs, like dysuria, frequency, urgency, rectal and/or perineal and/or suprapubic pain, acute swelling of the prostate, bladder neck spasms, and in some cases, acute urinary retention.

The diagnostic workup for ABP cannot include a number of key microbiological tests and imaging procedures that are necessary to confirm a diagnosis of CBP or CP/CPPS, as prostatic massage and transrectal ultrasound are at risk of worsening the infection and triggering urosepsis. For these reasons, the procedures to identify the causative pathogens of ABP are usually limited to midstream urine cultures. Blood cultures (BC) are sometimes necessary to detect the septic spread of the disease. A study by Etienne and coworkers demonstrated that a temperature above the 38.4 °C (101 °F) threshold could be significantly predictive of positive blood cultures [15]. Interestingly, the same study evidenced that patients with positive blood cultures showed nonsignificantly different death rates (positive BC: 4 %; negative BC: 3 %; $p=0.9$) and bacteriological failure rates (positive BC: 13 %; negative BC: 12 %; $p>0.9$), when compared to patients with negative blood cultures [15]. However, patients with positive cultures required longer hospitalization (positive BC: 10.3 days; negative BC: 9.2 days; $p=0.05$), showed longer duration of fever (positive BC: 3.7 days; negative BC: 2.8 days; $p<0.001$), and required significantly longer courses of antibacterial treatment (42 days versus 33 days, $p=0.05$).

Recommended therapy for ABP is mainly based on parenteral administration of full doses of bactericidal agents like fluoroquinolones (e.g., levofloxacin, ciprofloxacin), or third-generation cephalosporins (groups 3a/3b, e.g., cefodizime, cefotaxime, ceftriaxone, cefoperazone, ceftazidime). Beta-lactams can be combined with aminoglycosides (e.g., netilmicin, gentamicin, amikacin) to exploit the well-known synergic effects of these agents. When fever and other systemic signs or symptoms subside, therapy can be switched to oral antibacterials (most commonly fluoroquinolones, e.g., ciprofloxacin 500 mg twice daily, levofloxacin, 500–750 mg/day) for two or more weeks, to complete pathogen eradication and to lower the risk of chronicization of the infection. In less severe cases of ABP, not requiring intravenous treatment, oral fluoroquinolones may be administered for 10–14 days or longer (EAU guidelines: http://uroweb.org/wp-content/uploads/19-Urological-infections_LR.pdf). Lipsky and coworkers have published a comprehensive list of possible therapeutic options for ABP [33].

6.2 Chronic Bacterial Prostatitis

Category II chronic bacterial prostatitis (CBP) presents as a syndrome encompassing a characteristic array of signs/symptoms, including irritative and/or obstructive symptoms, perineal and suprapubic pain, other forms of pelvic and lumbar pain, painful ejaculation and sexual dysfunction, among others. Besides patient interview, clinical history, and urological visits, a number of diagnostic procedures are performed to complete the diagnosis of this disease. These include symptom-scoring questionnaires (the NIH-Chronic Prostatitis Symptom Index), transrectal prostate ultrasound, and culture of urethral, midstream, and post-massage urine and expressed prostatic secretions collected during standard segmented tests of the lower urinary tract [59].

According to the official NIH definition, category II CBP occurs when patients experience recurrent episodes of bacterial urinary tract infection caused by the same organism, usually *E. coli*, another gram-negative organism, or *Enterococcus* spp. Between symptomatic episodes of bacteriuria, lower urinary tract cultures can be used to document an infected prostate gland as the focus of these recurrent infections [27]. Thus, according to this definition, a *history* of repeated symptomatic episodes qualifies a prostatic infection as CBP and allows differential diagnosis between CBP and CP/CPPS.

Notably, this concept has not been unanimously and dogmatically applied in clinical practice, and a number of clinicians and scientists have maintained that the presence of pathogens in the post-massage urine or prostatic secretions of symptomatic patients may be etiologically linked to the clinical manifestation of category II CBP, even in the absence of a long, documented history of repeated flare-ups of the infection. According to this view, a *single*, nonfebrile, *persistently symptomatic* episode of clinical prostatitis with evidence of uropathogens in the prostate may represent a phase in a history of CBP, and there is therefore a requirement for it to be diagnosed and treated accordingly. Notably, antibacterial treatment of patients lacking such a documented history has been associated with symptom remission in numerous cases (e.g., [39]), suggesting that repeated flare-ups of the symptomatic infection are not an exclusive requirement of CBP.

6.2.1 Antibacterial Agents Recommended for Treatment of Chronic Bacterial Prostatitis: Pharmacological Considerations

According to international guidelines (e.g., EAU guidelines: http://uroweb.org/wp-content/uploads/19-Urological-infections_LR.pdf; UK guidelines: www.bashh.org/documents/1844.doc; Canadian guidelines: https://www.cua.org/themes/web/assets/files/guidelines/en/1121__1_.pdf; PERG-UK guidelines: http://prostatecanceruk.org/media/2491363/pcuk-chronic-prostatitis-guideline-full-feb-2015.pdf), an extended course (at least 4–6 weeks) of oral fluoroquinolone (FQ) therapy (e.g., ciprofloxacin 500 mg twice daily, levofloxacin 500–750 mg/day) is the established first-line therapeutic approach to CBP. Ideally, prior to therapy initiation, the causative pathogen ought to be isolated, and sensitivity to FQs should be unambiguously documented. It should also be considered that often the causative pathogens of CBP are strong biofilm producers and that this feature should be taken into consideration when a therapeutic protocol is being designed [4]. Fluoroquinolones target a broad spectrum of gram-negative and gram-positive bacteria, with later-generation compounds being more active against the latter and slightly less against the former. Ciprofloxacin remains among the most active antipseudomonal fluoroquinolones. In case of infection caused by anaerobic pathogens, the choice should be oriented toward FQs more active against these organisms, like levofloxacin. Off-label administration of potent, lipophilic anti-anaerobic agents like moxifloxacin may be considered in special cases, but the potential risk of renal or cardiological complications should be documented prior to initiation of therapy.

Resistance rates to fluoroquinolones are a primary matter of concern. One particularly worrisome determinant of FQ resistance is represented by the aminoglycoside acetyltransferase (AAC) encoded by the *aac (6')-Ib-cr* bacterial gene, already reported in uropathogen isolates in Denmark, the United Kingdom, the Netherlands, Germany, Switzerland, Hungary, Portugal, France, Spain, Italy, Slovenia, and Bulgaria [10, 11, 60].

The *aac (6')-Ib-cr* gene is a very interesting aspect of adaptive selection of bacterial resistance. This enzyme confers to uropathogenic *E. coli* or other *Enterobacteriaceae* a resistance to aminoglycoside antibiotics through acetylation (starting from acetyl-CoA) of specific NH2 residues at the level of amino sugars in molecules such as kanamycin, tobramycin, and amikacin.

It has been discovered that this acetyltransferase, in mutated form, is also able to confer resistance to certain fluoroquinolones. Figure 6.1 shows an acetylation reaction, catalyzed by AAC, of a (=NH) moiety within the piperazine ring of ciprofloxacin. This reaction changes significantly the structure of the drug and decreases by fourfold the susceptibility of pathogens to it [51].

Although the levels of resistance conferred by AAC are modest, the combined effect of AAC and the major resistance determinant qnrA can generate high levels of resistance to ciprofloxacin (MIC: 0.008 mg/L [WT *E. coli*]; 0.25 mg/L [only qnr in *E. coli*], 1 mg/L [qnr plus aac (6')-Ib-cr in *E. coli*]) [51].

Of equal importance is the effect exerted by AAC on the fluoroquinolone mutant prevention concentration (MPC) (up to 16-fold increase: $0.2 \rightarrow 3.2$ mg/L), which facilitates the survival of target site mutants [10, 51].

As described above, the acetyltransferase encoded by the gene *aac (6')-Ib-cr* induces resistance to fluoroquinolones through the modification of the =NH piperazine residue of drugs like ciprofloxacin or norfloxacin. Interestingly, the FQ levofloxacin has a methylated piperazine residue (Fig. 6.1), which is virtually protected from the action of AAC. This cannot only prevent the emergence of resistance in pathogens carrying the *aac (6')-Ib-cr* gene, but does not allow the combined effect of *aac (6')-Ib-cr* and *QnrA*, nor the increase of the MPC in exposed pathogens. Thus, where resistance rates caused by the AAC are present or suspected (e.g., in case of an antibiogram reporting a gram-negative pathogen intermediate resistant to ciprofloxacin but not to levofloxacin), levofloxacin, or other "protected" FQs like prulifloxacin or pefloxacin, may be considered [8, 20, 21].

In the case of fluoroquinolone resistance in non-multidrug-resistant strains, or in the presence of adverse reactions to FQs (e.g., tendonitis, phototoxicity, ECG-QT interval elongation), or in patients at high risk for these reactions, alternative agents like trimethoprim (or the co-trimoxazole combination) can be administered orally

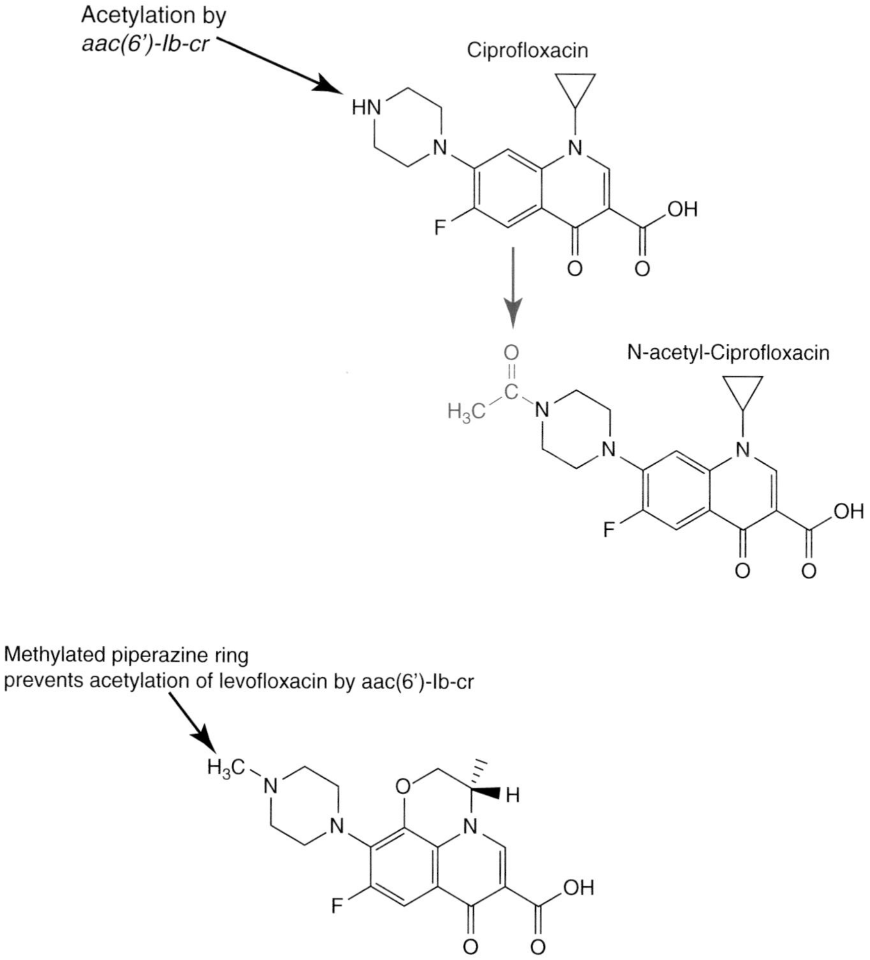

Acetylation by
aac(6')-Ib-cr

Ciprofloxacin

N-acetyl-Ciprofloxacin

Methylated piperazine ring
prevents acetylation of levofloxacin by aac(6')-Ib-cr

Fig. 6.1 An acetylation reaction, catalyzed by the enzyme *aac (6')-Ib-cr*, of the (=NH) moiety within the piperazine ring of ciprofloxacin. Levofloxacin (*bottom*) possesses a methylated piperazine residue (indicated by the *arrow*), virtually protecting the molecule from N-acetylation reactions

for a period of 12 weeks after the initial diagnosis. Notably, co-trimoxazole should be administered only in areas where resistance rates for *E. coli/Enterobacteriaceae* are inferior to 20 %. The patient should then be reassessed and therapy only continued if pretreatment cultures are still positive and the patient has reported positive effects from the treatment (EAU guidelines: http://uroweb.org/wp-content/uploads/19-Urological-infections_LR.pdf). Other drugs that may be considered in these cases are tetracyclines (e.g., doxycycline) and macrolides (e.g., azithromycin), though none of these agents is active against *P. aeruginosa*. Notably, administration of macrolides, alone or in combination with other antibacterials [37], may represent a convenient therapeutic option due to the optimal prostatic penetration of these agents; their activity against *S. aureus, C. trachomatis,* and anaerobes; their marked anti-biofilm activity; and their interesting immunomodulatory capacity. However, it should be emphasized that *Enterococci* are not sensitive to macrolides, and gram-negative pathogens show variable response to these agents.

Trimethoprim, tetracyclines, and macrolides have a good safety profile. However, certain macrolides can elongate the QT interval of the electrocardiogram [23] and should not be administered to patients at risk for polymorphic ventricular tachycardias.

In case of prostatic infections involving anaerobic protozoa like *Trichomonas vaginalis* or certain FQ-resistant anaerobic bacteria, a therapy with 500-mg metronidazole twice daily may be attempted, though this suggestion is only based on reports of single successful cases [1].

Like any therapeutic agent, antibacterials are subject to the laws of pharmacokinetics, describing the processes of drug absorption, blood-borne tissue distribution, metabolic transformation, and excretion.

Absorption of fluoroquinolones is generally optimal. The oral bioavailability (i.e., the fraction F of an oral dose that can actually reach the systemic circulation) of FQs is very high and most agents in this family show F levels of 90 % or higher. Other drugs used to treat chronic forms of bacterial prostatitis, like trimethoprim and doxycycline, also show excellent oral bioavailability ($F > 95$ %), whereas macrolides like azithromycin or clarithromycin show lower and variable absorption and bioavailability, ranging between 30 and 50 %.

Renal excretion of the unmodified drug (or of its active metabolites) is an essential characteristic of antibacterials that must be administered for treatment of urological infections like pyelonephritis or cystitis. This feature is not strictly required from drugs used to treat acute or chronic prostatitis, as these agents are distributed to the infected ducts of the gland via the prostate vasculature. Distribution of antibacterial agents to the ductal sites of infection in the prostate is indeed a critical issue, often affecting the success of treatment and greatly restricting the available therapeutic armamentarium. In order to reach infected ducts, a drug must cross the membranes of capillary endothelial cells, thus reaching the intracellular spaces and fluids of the gland parenchyma. Noncellular stromal components, the gland basement membrane, and different cell types (smooth-muscle cells, fibroblasts, etc.) may represent additional elements impeding the diffusion of antibacterial agents toward infected prostatic ducts (Fig. 6.2). However, the most critical obstacle to such diffusion process is represented by the presence of a putative "blood-prostate barrier."

6.2.2 A Blood-Prostate Barrier?

Successful antibacterial therapy leading ultimately to the cure of CBP has always been hindered by the fact that a large number of commonly used antibiotics, including almost all penicillins and cephalosporins, have proven, with very few exceptions [12] to be ineffective against sensitive uropathogens colonizing prostate glands and

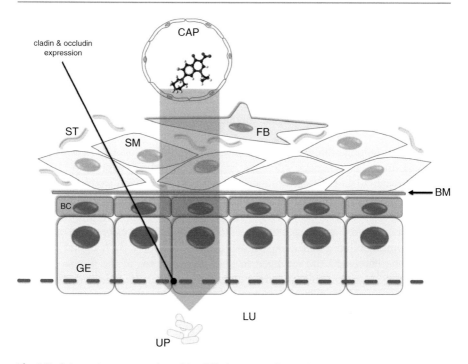

Fig. 6.2 Schematic representation of the diffusion route of an antibacterial agent (in this example: ciprofloxacin) from capillary vessels to pathogens colonizing a prostate ductal or luminal region. *BC* basal cell, *BM* basement membrane, *CAP* capillary vessel, *FB* fibroblast, *GE* glandular epithelium, *LU* lumen of gland or duct, *SM* smooth-muscle cell, *ST* noncellular stromal matrix components, *UP* infecting uropathogens. The *dashed red line* represents the putative barrier activity of tight junctions in the upper pole of columnar luminal cells; the *green arrow* shows the direction of the diffusion/distribution route

ducts. This evidence represents the *functional* and *empirical* demonstration of the presence of a "barrier activity" or "fence activity" within the prostate gland, preventing the distribution of blood-borne antibacterial agents to the site of infection. This barrier/fence activity is commonly referred to as the "blood-prostate barrier."

Barriers aimed at protecting gametes, embryos, and fetuses from external insults are well known and well described in humans as well as in animals. Blood-testis/blood-epididymis and ovarian blood-follicle barriers are typical examples of such structures. However, a comprehensive and systematic investigation aimed at demonstrating the presence and ultimate structure in humans of a blood-prostate barrier at the anatomical and ultrastructural levels has not been performed so far, to the authors' knowledge.

Nevertheless, there is sufficient evidence at the molecular level to support the hypothesis that a "barrier activity" or "fence activity" may indeed impede the access of a number of antibacterial agents to the lumen of prostate acini or ducts. Such evidence emerged from studies aimed at demonstrating the loss of cell-to-cell connections during the neoplastic transformation of the prostate, enabling cells showing increasingly malignant phenotypes to detach from the primary mass, infiltrate the underlying tissues, and eventually metastasize. In particular, a number of studies focused on the major structural components of tight junctions. Tight junctions (TJs) are closely associated membranes of adjacent cells, joining together to form a barrier which is virtually impermeable to water and many solutes, including most drugs. For example, tight junctions connecting capillary endothelial cells in the central nervous system are the fundamental components of the blood-brain barrier.

Occludins, and the family of claudin proteins, are the major constituents of tight junctions. Bush and coworkers demonstrated that occludin is expressed in normal human prostate glands [7] and shows a characteristic occlusion staining pattern in the apical region of secretory luminal cells. Together with occludin, claudins are the most important components of TJs, and form the paracellular barrier controlling the flux of ions and small molecules through the intercellular spaces between epithelial cells. By immunofluorescence experiments, claudins 1, 3, 4, 5, 7, 8, and 10 were shown to be expressed and arranged in junctional patterns in the mouse prostate epithelium [52], and an effective barrier activity, completely blocking the passage of blood-borne radiolabeled dextran to ductal fluids, was functionally demonstrated in the rat ventral prostate [17]. In humans, claudins 1, 3, 4, 5, and 7 were shown to be expressed and organized in junctional patterns in the apical region of columnar luminal cells in normal, nonneoplastic prostatic epithelia both in prostate cancer patients and in subjects affected by benign prostatic hyperplasia [3, 55, 61] (Fig. 6.2).

The fact that most studies demonstrated junctional patterns of expression of claudins and occludin in the apex region of luminal cells of the prostate glandular epithelium does not restrict the role of "barrier" or "fence" to these cells alone. For example, El-Alfy and coworkers have shown that basal cells within prostate glands, present in an even proportion (~1:1) with luminal cells only in humans, show a strict intercellular continuity ensured by the presence of junction-like complexes, which may indeed further contribute to the "barrier effect" elicited by tight junctions in the apex of luminal cells [14]. In addition, claudin-1 was shown to be preferentially expressed in basal cells in normal human prostates, thus confirming the presence of junctional structures also in deeper, non-apical cellular layers of prostate glands [26].

In summary, molecular evidence supports the hypothesis that adjacent epithelial cells in the prostate gland may be tightly connected to exert a barrier activity, preventing blood-borne drugs to reach the glandular lumen and to target the sites of pathogen colonization and infection. Notably, the presence of tight junction components in the human prostate has been established enough to prompt investigation of claudins 3 and 4 as potential therapeutic targets of cytotoxic *C. perfringens* enterotoxin, for therapy of primary and metastatic prostate cancer [35]. Moreover, several authors have proposed the use of microbubble-enhanced ultrasound in order to disrupt tight junctions and the "barrier activity" preventing efficient delivery of antibacterials to the lumen of prostate glands. Interesting results have been obtained so far in animal models [34, 54].

To circumvent this barrier activity at the glandular level within the prostate, lipophilic antibacterial agents, able to cross lipid cellular membranes by simple diffusion, must be used in order to achieve drug concentrations sufficient to eradicate the causative pathogens at the site of infection and to prevent the emergence of chemoresistant bacterial strains. In this respect, it was shown that more lipophilic fluoroquinolones like moxifloxacin can achieve higher concentrations in prostatic secretions, compared to less lipophilic molecules like norfloxacin or ciprofloxacin [47, 64].

When chronic infection is caused by intracellular pathogens replicating within luminal and basal cells of the prostate gland (e.g., *Chlamydia trachomatis*, but also various facultative intracellular bacteria), a therapy with drugs unable to efficiently reach the gland lumen may be attempted, as these agents do not need to cross the junctional barrier located in the apical region of the secretory epithelium to exert their effect. In this respect, macrolides show excellent intracellular penetration and are very effective anti-chlamydial agents in patients affected by chronic prostatitis [36, 58].

6.2.3   Management of Resistant Infections in the Superbug Era: Which Options for Chronic Bacterial Prostatitis?

Global surveillance studies indicate that fluoroquinolone resistance rates are rising dramatically in almost all bacterial species [13]. In some parts of the world, FQ resistance is increasing in *Enterobacteriaceae* causing community-acquired or healthcare-associated urinary tract infections, as well as sexually transmitted conditions, and in Asia, resistance levels over 50 % are commonly found.

For example, resistance rates to antibacterials in *Neisseria gonorrhoeae* can be as high as ~100 %, particularly in Asia; similar to tuberculosis, gonorrhea is nowadays categorized as "multidrug resistant," "extensively drug resistant," and "untreatable" [62].

On this basis, guidelines are being adapted worldwide, and alternative protocols are being tentatively suggested, until new studies confirm these indications, or new agents are discovered [41].

In the worrisome era of "superbugs" [9], what are the possible available alternatives to quinolones for managing the diseases treated in this chapter, and in particular CBP?

Indeed, the available armamentarium appears to be quite restricted, and evidence from randomized or cohort-observational studies is lacking. For a limited number of drugs, only published case reports or small patient series are available, and many agents must be administered off-label due to the lack of officially approved and registered indications for prostatitis.

For CBP caused by *gram-negative pathogens*, carbapenems and aminoglycosides, alone or in combination, are possible alternatives to FQs.

The prostate penetration of meropenem has been documented, and sufficient bactericidal concentrations are achieved in the prostate tissue for most pathogens, albeit the antipseudomonal activity of this drug in the prostate is uncertain [44].

For few aminoglycosides (e.g., netilmicin in some European countries), "prostatitis" is an approved indication, and administration is on-label. Adoption of aminoglycosides for long-term treatment of CBP can be hampered by the risk of toxicity to the kidneys and to the inner ear. Whereas renal damage can be sometimes reversible and may be in part avoidable through careful monitoring and continuous patient hydration, cochleotoxicity and/or vestibulotoxicity can appear abruptly and be severe, leading in some cases to profound, irreversible sensorineural hearing loss [46]. The discovery in the late 1990s of the adenine-guanine substitution at the 1555th nucleotide of mitochondrial DNA as the responsible of the onset of hearing loss, often after the very first dose of aminoglycoside [49], was a major scientific breakthrough, and today pharmacogenetic testing for A1555G, C1494T, and other ototoxicity-predisposing mutations may be performed prior to aminoglycoside therapy [6, 63]. In this regard, the Sanford Guide to Antimicrobial Therapy (Table 10A Antibiotic Dosage and Side-Effects) warns clinicians that one in 500 European patients may have mitochondrial mutations that predict cochlear toxicity [22]. Hence, if pharmacogenetic testing is not feasible, careful exclusion of a history of matrilineal deafness is a strongly recommended assessment prior to aminoglycoside administration.

A drug that may be potentially active in the management of a gram-negative prostatic infection is fosfomycin, administered intravenously or orally; evidence of successful resolution of CBP cases was recently presented, though further investigation is warranted [18, 25].

The emergence of enterococcal and staphylococcal strains with multidrug-resistant ability has greatly complicated the management of prostatic infections, and there is an urgent need to assess the efficacy of alternative agents in the frame of adequately designed, powered, and controlled clinical studies. At present (year 2015), the published evidence is scant, and only case reports and case studies are available. For this reason, any recommendation or suggestion is only tentative and based on limited empirical/anecdotal experience.

Gram-positive pathogens like *Enterococcus faecalis*, *Enterococcus faecium*, and *Staphylococcus aureus* (methicillin resistant) are generally sensitive to agents like linezolid and tigecycline.

The oxazolidinone linezolid is officially indicated for treatment of skin, soft tissue, and lung infections, though its activity against fluoroquinolone-resistant uropathogens has been investigated [45, 65]. Linezolid is bacteriostatic against *enterococci* and *staphylococci*, but bactericidal for *streptococci*. It can be administered orally or parenterally, shows a bioavailability of almost 100 %, and the distribution volume equals approximately the total body water (~40 L). The half-life is about 5–7 h, and twice-daily administration is advised [2, 48]. Metabolic acidosis and myelosuppression are among the more severe adverse effects caused by the drug, though in a limited number of cases. Linezolid, administered intravenously (600 mg, twice daily), in combination with oral co-trimoxazole (960 mg b.i.d.), was effective in resolving a complicated case of prostatitis, likely involving both *Enterococci* and various *Enterobacteriaceae* [50].

Tigecycline, a glycylcycline structurally resembling tetracycline, can be used to treat gram-positive, but also gram-negative (including metallo-β-Lactamase multidrug-resistant *Enterobacteriaceae*, but not *P. aeruginosa* or *Proteus spp.*) and anaerobic bacterial infections. It is mainly bacteriostatic, but in few cases it is bactericidal, depending on the targeted organism. Its high volume of distribution of 7–10 L/kg suggests diffuse tissue penetration. Moreover, the drug has a conveniently long half-life (about 40 h). A comprehensive analysis of the potential activity of this agent against CBP, together with a detailed case report, has been published by Bates and coworkers [5]. These authors describe administration of intravenous tigecycline, 50 mg twice daily, after a single "kick-in" 100-mg dose, for 6 weeks.

Among agents active against gram-positive pathogens, the anti-mycobacterial agent rifampicin had been shown to be effective against CBP caused by *S. aureus* and may be considered for treatment of fluoroquinolone-resistant, MRSA [19]. Moreover, lipoglycopeptides like dalbavancin and oritavancin are active against MRSA and VRE, have very long plasma half-lives, and are particularly active against biofilm-embedded pathogens. The activity of these interesting drugs in CBP is not yet established. Data are also awaited to confirm preliminary anecdotal reports of the efficacy of piperacillin/tazobactam against complicated cases of enterococcal CBP.

6.3   Chronic Prostatitis/Chronic Pelvic Pain Syndrome (CP/CPPS) with *Bacterial Component*: A New Disease Category?

Category III CP/CPPS, with its inflammatory (IIIa) and non-inflammatory (IIIb) variants, has been originally defined [27], diagnosed, and investigated [42] as a prostatitis syndrome involving pelvic pain and voiding symptoms in the presence of *sterile* microbiological cultures of expressed prostatic secretions and/or urine specimens following prostatic massage. Over time, this definition has evolved, and experts have proposed a model whereby the prostate of patients with CP/CPPS may be colonized by a variety of organisms, including the etiological agents of acute and chronic bacterial prostatitis (*E. coli*, *Klebsiella spp.*, other *Enterobacteriaceae*, *Enterococci*) but also by other pathogens like *Chlamydia trachomatis* and *Mycoplasmata* [56, 57]. This model points to the controversial concept of "bacterial CP/CPPS" (see answer to: [38]). According to some authors, these bacteria may not act as single etiological determinants in category III CP/CPPS, but constitute a "bystander flora," whose pharmacological eradication may or may not result in complete or partial symptom remission. This concept has led to the inclusion of an infection component into the UPOINT algorithm, a system recently proposed to improve the phenotypic profiling and the symptom-directed treatment of patients with CP/CPPS, addressing the urinary, psychosocial, organ specific, infection, neurological, and tenderness domains of the disease [43]. Whereas some authors failed to demonstrate the influence of pathogens isolated from prostate-specific specimens on CP/CPPS clinical symptoms [56], others found that the presence of microorganisms may influence the severity of clinical symptoms of CP/CPPS in UPOINT-phenotyped patients. In a cohort of 937 individuals, predominantly second referral Italian patients with evidence of infection at the prostatic level, total NIH-CPSI symptom scores were significantly increased (~20 %), compared to patients showing a negative UPOINT infection domain [40]. Similarly, in a prospective study performed on a cohort of about 400 Chinese patients, it was shown that total NIH-CPSI symptom scores were increased by 20–25 % ($p < 0.05$, Mann-Whitney) in patients with a positive infection domain of the UPOINT system, compared to uninfected subjects [66].

These results suggest that the presence of pathogens in the prostate gland may exert a significant effect on the clinical presentation of patients affected by CP/CPPS and that a positive UPOINT infection domain can be a codeterminant of the severity of symptoms of CP/CPPS. In this case, antibacterial agents may be used for treating patients showing evidence of prostate colonization by uropathogens or by other suspiciously pathogenic bacteria. In fact, administration of antibacterial agents to CP/CPPS patients is part of the UPOINT therapeutic algorithm. In this case, the same pharmacokinetic criteria directing the choice of appropriate agents for management of cat. II CBP may apply to antibacterial treatment of cat. III CP/CPPS. International guidelines indicate that a fluoroquinolone should be given for at least 4 weeks. In case of fluoroquinolone resistance, oral trimethoprim may be administered for a period of 4–12 weeks after the initial diagnosis (EAU guidelines: http://uroweb.org/wp-content/uploads/19-Urological-infections_LR.pdf).

6.4   Mycobacterial Prostatitis

Twenty percent of patients with tuberculosis (TB) will develop an extrapulmonary manifestation of the disease over time, the most common site of infection being the urogenital tract. Tuberculosis of the urogenital tract is the second most common form of TB in countries where the disease is epidemic (e.g., India, China), the third most common form in regions where the prevalence of the disease is low, and has been reported to be steadily increasing worldwide in patients suffering from acquired immunodeficiency syndrome [16, 32].

Prostate tuberculosis (PTB), sometimes also referred to as *granulomatous prostatitis*, due to the appearance of typical granulomas mainly in the peripheral zone of the gland in patients with mycobacterial infection, is known to be a rare occurrence, though such rarity is difficult to understand in view of the almost constant exposure of the urethra to infected urine. In fact, according to Kulchavenya, PTB can be detected in 77 % of men dying from any form of tuberculosis [31]. Thus, it is likely that a number of cases of PTB are overlooked during the course of patients' medical history.

The possible patterns of spread of PTB include a descending infection from the kidney, direct intracanalicular extension from a neighboring tuberculous focus in the genital tract, or a hematogenous spread [24].

The pharmacological treatment of choice is chemotherapy using three or four anti-TB agents for up to 9–12 months [24, 28]. The results of therapy depend on the promptness of diagnosis, as patients diagnosed in late cavern stage are unlikely to be cured. Kulchavenya and Khomyakov showed that standard chemotherapy for PTB is only partially effective, since only 22.8 % of patients were found to be cured with regimens including isoniazid, rifampicin, pyrazinamide, and streptomycin, the disease becoming chronic and progressive in the remaining 77.2 % of cases [30]. However, a cohort study by the same research group has demonstrated that a pharmacological protocol based on isoniazid (10 mg/kg), pyrazinamide (25 mg/kg), streptomycin (1,000 mg intramuscular), rifampicin (10 mg/kg), and the fluoroquinolone ofloxacin (10 mg/kg), administered during the "intensive phase" of therapy and eventually switched to a rifampicin-isoniazid combination for 6 months, resulted in undetectable *Mycobacteria* and disappearance of pain, dysuria, and pyospermia in 78 % of cases [29]. Interestingly, this outcome could be achieved only in 44 % of control patients who received the same regimen not including ofloxacin [29]. Being PTB a rare disease, it is perhaps unrealistic to expect confirmation of these interesting results in a randomized setting. Nevertheless, the almost twofold increase in therapeutic success shown by the fluoroquinolone arm points to the relative robustness of this evidence.

References

1. Abdolrasouli A, Amin A, Baharsefat M, Roushan A, Mofidi S (2007) Persistent urethritis and prostatitis due to Trichomonas vaginalis: a case report. Can J Infect Dis Med Microbiol 18(5):308–310
2. Ament PW, Jamshed N, Horne JP (2002) Linezolid: its role in the treatment of gram-positive, drug-resistant bacterial infections. Am Fam Physician 65(4):663–670
3. Bartholow TL, Chandran UR, Becich MJ, Parwani AV (2011) Immunohistochemical profiles of claudin-3 in primary and metastatic prostatic adenocarcinoma. Diagn Pathol 6:12
4. Bartoletti R, Cai T, Nesi G, Albanese S, Meacci F, Mazzoli S, Naber K (2014) The impact of biofilm-producing bacteria on chronic bacterial prostatitis treatment: results from a longitudinal cohort study. World J Urol 32(3):737–742
5. Bates D, Parkins M, Hellweg R, Gibson K, Bugar JM (2012) Tigecycline treatment of urinary tract infection and prostatitis: case report and literature review. Can J Hosp Pharm 65(3):209–215
6. Bitner-Glindzicz M, Pembrey M, Duncan A, Heron J, Ring SM, Hall A, Rahman S (2009) Prevalence of mitochondrial 1555A–>G mutation in European children. N Engl J Med 360(6):640–642
7. Busch C, Hanssen TA, Wagener C, OBrink B (2002) Down-regulation of CEACAM1 in human prostate cancer: correlation with loss of cell polarity, increased proliferation rate, and Gleason grade 3 to 4 transition. Hum Pathol 33(3):290–298
8. Cai T, Mazzoli S, Bechi A, Addonisio P, Mondaini N, Pagliai RC, Bartoletti R (2009) Serenoa repens associated with Urtica dioica (ProstaMEV) and curcumin and quercitin (FlogMEV) extracts are able to improve the efficacy of prulifloxacin in bacterial prostatitis patients: results from a prospective randomised study. Int J Antimicrob Agents 33(6):549–553
9. Casey G (2012) Antibiotics and the rise of superbugs. Nurs N Z 18(10):20–24
10. Cattoir V, Nordmann P (2009) Plasmid-mediated quinolone resistance in gram-negative bacterial species: an update. Curr Med Chem 16:1028–1046
11. Cerquetti M, Giufrè M, García-Fernández A, Accogli M, Fortini D, Luzzi I, Carattoli A (2010) Ciprofloxacin-resistant, CTX-M-15-producing Escherichia coli ST131 clone in extraintestinal infections in Italy. Clin Microbiol Infect 16:1555–1558

12. Charalabopoulos K, Karachalios G, Baltogiannis D, Charalabopoulos A, Giannakopoulos X, Sofikitis N (2003) Penetration of antimicrobial agents into the prostate. Chemotherapy 49(6):269–279
13. Dalhoff A (2012) Global fluoroquinolone resistance epidemiology and implications for clinical use. Interdiscip Perspect Infect Dis 2012:976273
14. El-Alfy M, Pelletier G, Hermo LS, Labrie F (2000) Unique features of the basal cells of human prostate epithelium. Microsc Res Tech 51(5):436–446
15. Etienne M, Pestel-Caron M, Chapuzet C, Bourgeois I, Chavanet P, Caron F (2010) Should blood cultures be performed for patients with acute prostatitis? J Clin Microbiol 48(5):1935–1938
16. Figueiredo AA, Lucon AM (2008) Urogenital tuberculosis: update and review of 8961 cases from the world literature. Rev Urol 10(3):207–217
17. Fulmer BR, Turner TT (2000) A blood-prostate barrier restricts cell and molecular movement across the rat ventral prostate epithelium. J Urol 163(5):1591–1594
18. Gardiner BJ, Mahony AA, Ellis AG, Lawrentschuk N, Bolton DM, Zeglinski PT, Frauman AG, Grayson ML (2014) Is fosfomycin a potential treatment alternative for multidrug-resistant gram-negative prostatitis? Clin Infect Dis 58(4):e101–e105
19. Giamarellou H, Kosmidis J, Leonidas M, Papadakis M, Daikos GK (1982) A study of the effectiveness of rifaprim in chronic prostatitis caused mainly by Staphylococcus aureus. J Urol 128(2):321–324
20. Giannarini G, Mogorovich A, Valent F, Morelli G, De Maria M, Manassero F, Barbone F, Selli C (2007) Prulifloxacin versus levofloxacin in the treatment of chronic bacterial prostatitis: a prospective, randomized, double-blind trial. J Chemother 19(3):304–308, PubMed
21. Giannopoulos A, Koratzanis G, Giamarellos-Bourboulis EJ, Stinios I, Chrisofos M, Giannopoulou M, Giamarellou H (2001) Pharmacokinetics of intravenously administered pefloxacin in the prostate; perspectives for its application in surgical prophylaxis. Int J Antimicrob Agents 17(3):221–224
22. Gilbert DN (2013) The Sanford guide to antimicrobial therapy. Antimicrobial Therapy, Sperryville
23. Guo D, Cai Y, Chai D, Liang B, Bai N, Wang R (2010) The cardiotoxicity of macrolides: a systematic review. Pharmazie 65(9):631–640
24. Gupta N, Mandal AK, Singh SK (2008) Tuberculosis of the prostate and urethra: a review. Indian J Urol 24(3):388–391
25. Hagiya H, Ninagawa M, Hasegawa K, Terasaka T, Kimura K, Waseda K, Hanayama Y, Sendo T, Otsuka F (2014) Fosfomycin for the treatment of prostate infection. Intern Med 53(22):2643–2646
26. Krajewska M, Olson AH, Mercola D, Reed JC, Krajewski S (2007) Claudin-1 immunohistochemistry for distinguishing malignant from benign epithelial lesions of prostate. Prostate 67(9):907–910
27. Krieger JN, Nyberg L Jr, Nickel JC (1999) NIH consensus definition and classification of prostatitis. JAMA 282(3):236–237
28. Kulchavenya E (2013) Best practice in the diagnosis and management of urogenital tuberculosis. Ther Adv Urol 5(3):143–151
29. Kulchavenya E, Brizhatyuk E, Khomyakov V (2014) Diagnosis and therapy for prostate tuberculosis. Ther Adv Urol 6(4):129–134
30. Kulchavenya E, Khomyakov V (2006) Male genital tuberculosis in Siberians. World J Urol 24(1):74–78
31. Kulchavenya E, Kim CS, Bulanova O, Zhukova I (2012) Male genital tuberculosis: epidemiology and diagnostic. World J Urol 30(1):15–21
32. Lenk S, Schroeder J (2001) Genitourinary tuberculosis. Curr Opin Urol 11(1):93–98
33. Lipsky BA, Byren I, Hoey CT (2010) Treatment of bacterial prostatitis. Clin Infect Dis 50(12):1641–1652

34. Liu Y, Yi S, Zhang J, Fang Z, Zhou F, Jia W, Liu Z, Ye G (2013) Effect of microbubble-enhanced ultrasound on prostate permeability: a potential therapeutic method for prostate disease. Urology 81(4):921.e1–7
35. Maeda T, Murata M, Chiba H, Takasawa A, Tanaka S, Kojima T, Masumori N, Tsukamoto T, Sawada N (2012) Claudin-4-targeted therapy using Clostridium perfringens enterotoxin for prostate cancer. Prostate 72(4):351–360
36. Magri V, Marras E, Skerk V, Markotić A, Restelli A, Garlaschi MC, Perletti G (2010) Eradication of Chlamydia trachomatis parallels symptom regression in chronic bacterial prostatitis patients treated with a fluoroquinolone-macrolide combination. Andrologia 42(6):366–375
37. Magri V, Montanari E, Škerk V, Markotić A, Marras E, Restelli A, Naber KG, Perletti G (2011) Fluoroquinolone-macrolide combination therapy for chronic bacterial prostatitis: retrospective analysis of pathogen eradication rates, inflammatory findings and sexual dysfunction. Asian J Androl 13:819–827
38. Magri V, Perletti G (2008) Re: How does the pre-massage and post-massage 2-glass test compare to the meares-stamey 4-glass test in men with chronic prostatitis/chronic pelvic pain syndrome? J. C. Nickel, D. Shoskes, Y. Wang, R. B. Alexander, J. E. Fowler, jr., S. Zeitlin, M. P. O'Leary,M. A. Pontari, A. J. Schaeffer, J. R. Landis, L. Nyberg, J. W. Kusek and K. J. Propert J Urol 2006; 176: 119–124. J Urol 180(4):1571–1572
39. Magri V, Trinchieri A, Pozzi G, Restelli A, Garlaschi MC, Torresani E, Zirpoli P, Marras E, Perletti G (2007) Efficacy of repeated cycles of combination therapy for the eradication of infecting organisms in chronic bacterial prostatitis. Int J Antimicrob Agents 29(5):549–556
40. Magri V, Wagenlehner F, Perletti G, Schneider S, Marras E, Naber KG, Weidner W (2010) Use of the UPOINT chronic prostatitis/chronic pelvic pain syndrome classification in European patient cohorts: sexual function domain improves correlations. J Urol 184:2339–2345
41. Marino Sabo E, Stern JJ (2014) Approach to antimicrobial prophylaxis for urology procedures in the era of increasing fluoroquinolone resistance. Ann Pharmacother 48(3):380–386
42. Nickel JC, Downey J, Johnston B, Clark J, Canadian Prostatitis Research Group (2001) Predictors of patient response to antibiotic therapy for the chronic prostatitis/chronic pelvic pain syndrome: a prospective multicenter clinical trial. J Urol 165(5):1539–1544
43. Nickel JC, Shoskes D (2009) Phenotypic approach to the management of chronic prostatitis/chronic pelvic pain syndrome. Curr Urol Rep 10(4):307–312
44. Nishikawa G, Ikawa K, Nakamura K, Yamada Y, Zennami K, Mitsui K, Narushima M, Ikeda K, Morikawa N, Sumitomo M (2013) Prostatic penetration of meropenem in humans, and dosage considerations for prostatitis based on a site-specific pharmacokinetic/pharmacodynamic evaluation. Int J Antimicrob Agents 41(3):267–271
45. Onda H, Wagenlehner FM, Lehn N, Naber KG (2001) In vitro activity of linezolid against gram-positive uropathogens of hospitalized patients with complicated urinary tract infections. Int J Antimicrob Agents 18(3):263–266
46. Perletti G, Vral A, Patrosso MC, Marras E, Ceriani I, Willems P, Fasano M, Magri V (2008) Prevention and modulation of aminoglycoside ototoxicity (review). Mol Med Rep 1(1):3–13
47. Perletti G, Wagenlehner FM, Naber KG, Magri V (2009) Enhanced distribution of fourth-generation fluoroquinolones in prostatic tissue. Int J Antimicrob Agents 33(3):206–210
48. Perry CM, Jarvis B (2001) Linezolid: a review of its use in the management of serious gram-positive infections. Drugs 61(4):525–551
49. Prezant TR, Agapian JV, Bohlman MC, Bu X, Oztas S, Qiu WQ, Arnos KS, Cortopassi GA, Jaber L, Rotter JI, Shohat M, Fischel-Ghodsian N (1993) Mitochondrial ribosomal RNA mutation associated with both antibiotic-induced and non-induced syndromic deafness. Nat Genet 4:289–294
50. Pronk MJ, Pelger RC, Baranski AG, van Dam A, Arend SM (2006) Cure of chronic prostatitis presumably due to Enterococcus spp and gram-negative bacteria. Eur J Clin Microbiol Infect Dis 25(4):270–271

51. Robicsek A, Strahilevitz J, Jacoby GA, Macielag M, Abbanat D, Park CH, Bush K, Hooper DC (2006) Fluoroquinolone-modifying enzyme: a new adaptation of a common aminoglycoside acetyltransferase. Nat Med 12:83–88
52. Sakai N, Chiba H, Fujita H, Akashi Y, Osanai M, Kojima T, Sawada N (2007) Expression patterns of claudin family of tight-junction proteins in the mouse prostate. Histochem Cell Biol 127(4):457–462
53. Santillo VM, Lowe FC (2006) The management of chronic prostatitis in men with HIV. Curr Urol Rep 7(4):313–319
54. Shang Y, Cui D, Yi S (2014) Opening tight junctions may be key to opening the blood-prostate barrier. Med Sci Monit 20:2504–2507
55. Sheehan GM, Kallakury BV, Sheehan CE, Fisher HA, Kaufman RP Jr, Ross JS (2007) Loss of claudins-1 and −7 and expression of claudins-3 and −4 correlate with prognostic variables in prostatic adenocarcinomas. Hum Pathol 38(4):564–569
56. Shoskes DA, Nickel JC, Dolinga R, Prots D (2009) Clinical phenotyping of patients with chronic prostatitis/chronic pelvic pain syndrome and correlation with symptom severity. Urology 73:538–542
57. Shoskes DA, Nickel JC, Rackley RR, Pontari MA (2009) Clinical phenotyping in chronic prostatitis/chronic pelvic pain syndrome and interstitial cystitis: a management strategy for urologic chronic pelvic pain syndromes. Prostate Cancer Prostatic Dis 12(2):177–183
58. Skerk V, Krhen I, Lisić M, Begovac J, Cajić V, Zekan S, Skerk V, Sternak SL, Topić A, Schönwald S (2004) Azithromycin: 4.5- or 6.0-gram dose in the treatment of patients with chronic prostatitis caused by Chlamydia trachomatis–a randomized study. J Chemother 16(4):408–410
59. Stamey TA (1981) Prostatitis. J R Soc Med 74(1):22–40
60. Strahilevitz J, Jacoby GA, Hooper DC, Robicsek A (2009) Plasmid-mediated quinolone resistance: a multifaceted threat. Clin Microbiol Rev 22:664–689
61. Swisshelm K, Machl A, Planitzer S, Robertson R, Kubbies M, Hosier S (1999) SEMP1, a senescence-associated cDNA isolated from human mammary epithelial cells, is a member of an epithelial membrane protein superfamily. Gene 226(2):285–295
62. Unemo M, Nicholas RA (2012) Emergence of multidrug-resistant, extensively drug-resistant and untreatable gonorrhea. Future Microbiol 7(12):1401–1422
63. Vandebona H, Mitchell P, Manwaring N, Griffiths K, Gopinath B, Wang JJ, Sue CM (2009) Prevalence of mitochondrial 1555A-> G mutation in adults of European descent. N Engl J Med 360(6):642–644
64. Wagenlehner FM, Kees F, Weidner W, Wagenlehner C, Naber KG (2008) Concentrations of moxifloxacin in plasma and urine, and penetration into prostatic fluid and ejaculate, following single oral administration of 400 mg to healthy volunteers. Int J Antimicrob Agents 31(1):21–26
65. Wagenlehner FM, Naber KG (2004) New drugs for gram-positive uropathogens. Int J Antimicrob Agents 24(Suppl 1):S39–S43
66. Zhao Z, Zhang J, He J, Zeng G (2013) Clinical utility of the UPOINT phenotype system in Chinese males with chronic prostatitis/chronic pelvic pain syndrome (CP/CPPS): a prospective study. PLoS One 8:e52044

Treatment of Nonbacterial Prostatitis: What's New?

7

Paolo Verze and Luca Venturino

7.1 Introduction

Chronic pain (CP) in the region of the prostate has been linked to the term "prostatitis" in the past, although there is a proven bacterial infection in only 10 % of the cases [1]. The remaining 90 % should be classified as prostate pain syndrome (PPS), based on the fact that there is no proven infection or other obvious pathology. PPS is defined as the occurrence of persistent or recurrent episodic pain over at least 3 out of the past 6 months (which is convincingly reproduced by prostate palpation), while there is no proven infection or other obvious local pathology.

PPS is often associated with negative cognitive, behavioral, sexual, or emotional consequences [2], as well as with symptoms suggestive of lower urinary tract and sexual dysfunction [3, 4].

As per the classification proposed by the National Institute of Diabetes and Digestive and Kidney Diseases (NIDDK), this condition correlates to CP/CPPS (cat. III). Laboratory diagnosis goes along with sterile specimen cultures and either significant or insignificant white blood cell counts in prostate-specific specimens (i.e., semen, expressed prostatic secretions, and urine collected after prostate massage) [5].

NIH definition for CP/CPPS differentiates two peculiar conditions based on the presence/absence of inflammatory indices (CP/CPPS categories: IIIa inflammatory or IIIb noninflammatory). At present, according to EAU guidelines, the only therapeutic consequence arising from differentiating inflammatory from noninflammatory PPS is that detection of an inflammatory white cell response provides a scientific rationale for tentative use of antibiotics. For the present purpose, however, the two forms of type III prostatitis are considered as one entity.

P. Verze (✉) • L. Venturino, MD
Department of Urology, University of Naples, Naples, Italy
e-mail: pverze@gmail.com

© Springer International Publishing Switzerland 2016
T. Cai, T.E. Bjerklund Johansen (eds.), *Prostatitis and Its Management: Concepts and Recommendations for Clinical Practice*, DOI 10.1007/978-3-319-25175-2_7

7.1.1 Epidemiological Data

There is only limited information on the true prevalence of PPS in the population. As a result of significant overlap of symptoms with other conditions (e.g., benign prostate syndrome (BPS)), purely symptom-based case definitions may not reflect the true prevalence of PPS [6, 7].

To date in the literature, numbers of the population-based prevalence of prostatitis symptoms are reported ranging from 1 to 14.2 % [8, 9]. Furthermore, there is evidence that the risk of prostatitis increases with age (men aged 50–59 years have a 3.1-fold greater risk than those aged 20–39 years).

7.2 Clinical Management of CP/CPPS

7.2.1 General Principles

Management of chronic pelvic pain syndrome (CPPS) is challenging. Our understanding of the etiology and pathogenesis of the condition remains inadequate, and current treatment strategies are frequently ineffective. Researchers and clinicians in the field generally agree that patients with CPPS are not a homogeneous entity presenting with pain arising in pelvic organs, but rather are individuals with widely different clinical phenotypes [10].

It is likely that different mechanisms and dynamics are the basis for the highly individual courses of these conditions.

In 2004, the EAU guidelines on chronic pelvic pain expert panel proposed for the first time a multidimensional approach to CPPS.

Shoskes et al. were the first to propose a clinical phenotype-based classification system with six domains: urinary, psychosocial, organ specific, infection, neurologic/systemic, and tenderness (UPOINT) (Fig. 7.1) [11]. UPOINT aims to improve the understanding and management of prostate and bladder pain syndromes, and the value of the system is that it will induce reflection on the multidimensional complexity of this group of conditions [12].

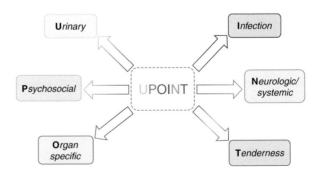

Fig. 7.1 UPOINT structure with the six domains

Successively, due to the high prevalence of sexual dysfunction in men with urological chronic pelvic pain syndrome, Magri et al. proposed the addition of a sexual dysfunction domain in regard to symptom correlation to the conventional UPOINT system (UPOINT-S) [13].

In another study, 162 men were assessed using UPOINT criteria and after adding the sexual dysfunction domain. Using multiple regression analysis UPOINT(S) criteria were then compared to quality of life, as measured by the SF-36® health outcome survey and Chronic Prostatitis Symptom Index. The total number of UPOINT(S) domains correlated with SF-36 and Chronic Prostatitis Symptom Index scores. Using regression analysis the two significant predictors of SF-36 scores were the psychosocial and sexual domains. Men with sexual dysfunction had significantly worse quality of life than men without the condition. Authors' conclusion was that adding a sexual dysfunction domain to UPOINT may help improve quality of life in men treated for urological chronic pelvic pain syndrome [14].

More recently, the US NIH/NIDDK launched and funded the Multidisciplinary Approach to Pelvic Pain (MAPP) research consortium program, aimed to better understand the pathophysiology of urological chronic pelvic pain syndromes (UCPPSs), to inform future clinical trials and improve clinical care. The primary scientific protocol for the Trans-MAPP Epidemiology/Phenotyping (EP) Study comprises a multisite, longitudinal observational study, including biweekly Internet-based symptom assessments, following a comprehensive in-clinic deep-phenotyping array of urological symptoms, non-urological symptoms, and psychosocial factors to evaluate men and women with UCPPS. Additional, complementary studies addressing diverse hypotheses are integrated into the Trans-MAPP EP Study to provide a systemic characterization of study participants, including biomarker discovery studies of infectious agents, quantitative sensory testing, and structural and resting-state neuroimaging and functional neurobiology studies. A highly novel effort to develop and assess clinically relevant animal models of UCPPS was also undertaken to allow improved translation between clinical and mechanistic studies. Another objective of MAPP is to achieve phenotyping of CPPS patients that could lead to individualized treatment strategies [15].

Based on this innovative classification system, there is growing evidence for advantage of an integrated team approach to assess and manage PPS patients. This is most likely to occur in specialized centers.

As a result of the multifactorial origin of PPS, one reason for treatment failure in some large randomized placebo-controlled trials may be the heterogeneity of the patient population. A prospective series of phenotypically directed treatment for PPS has shown significant improvement of symptoms and QoL [16]. Monotherapeutic strategies for the treatment of PPS may fail; therefore, most patients require multimodal treatment aimed at the main symptoms, taking comorbidity into account. In the past 10 years, results from RCTs have led to advances in standard and novel treatment options.

7.2.2 Treatment Modalities

Table 7.1 lists different therapeutic options according to UPOINT domains.

7.2.2.1 α-Blockers

α-Blockers act on CP/CPPS by relieving the smooth muscle spasm within the bladder neck and prostatic urethra, which eases urinary voiding. This class of drugs can be recommended as first-line medical therapy, particularly in α-blocker-naive men with moderately severe symptoms who have relatively recent onset of symptoms. α-Blockers cannot be recommended in men with long-standing CP/CPPS who have tried and failed α-blockers in the past.

Ten placebo-controlled RCTs ($n = 58–272$) were identified that evaluated alpha-adrenergic antagonists (tamsulosin [17, 18], alfuzosin [19, 20], doxazosin [21, 22], terazosin [23, 24], and silodosin [25]) in CBP and CP/CPPS.

Table 7.1 Therapeutic options according to UPOINT domains

UPOINT description	Suggested therapies
Urinary NIH-CPSI urinary score >4 Obstructive voiding symptoms Bothersome urgency, frequency, and/or nocturia Elevated post-void residual	Antimuscarinics α-Blockers
Psychosocial Clinical depression Evidence of maladaptive coping Anxiety/stress	Counseling Cognitive behavioral therapy Antidepressants Anxiolytics
Organ specific Specific prostate tenderness Leukocytosis in prostatic fluid Hematospermia Extensive prostatic calcification	α-Blockers 5-α-Reductase inhibitors Phytotherapy Prostate massage
Infection Gram-negative bacilli or enterococci localized to prostatic fluid[a] Documented successful response to antimicrobial therapy	Antimicrobials
Neurologic/systemic conditions Clinical evidence of central neuropathy Pain beyond pelvis Irritable bowel syndrome Fibromyalgia Chronic fatigue syndrome	Neuromodulators Specific therapies for associated conditions
Tenderness of skeletal muscles Palpable tenderness and/or painful muscle spasm or trigger points in abdomen and/or pelvic floor	Focused pelvic physiotherapy General physiotherapy Exercises

Adapted from Nickel [35]
NIH-CPSI National Institutes of Health Chronic Prostatitis Symptom Index, *UPOINT* Urinary, Psychosocial, Organ specific, Infection, Neurologic/systemic, and Tenderness
[a]Exclude patients with clinical category I or II prostatitis

The majority of the studies ($n = 8$) showed positive results, with significant differences vs. placebo in improving NIH-CPSI total, urinary symptom, pain, and/or QoL scores or in scores using other validated symptom scoring tools.

However, there was heterogeneity in primary end points, patient eligibility criteria (e.g., previous exposure to alpha-blockers), and trial duration (6 weeks–6 months). A recent systematic review and network meta-analysis of alpha-blocker RCTs found significant differences vs. placebo in improving total, pain, voiding, and QoL NIH-CPSI scores [26]. However, another recent systematic review questioned the clinical significance of these reductions [27]. Major limitations with regard to previously published studies were that two of the larger, placebo-controlled trials that evaluated tamsulosin ($n = 196$) [17] and alfuzosin ($n = 272$) [20] failed to show any significant difference in total NIH-CPSI scores, the only outcome achieving statistical significance being the score for ejaculation on the Male Sexual Health Questionnaire ($p = 0.04$) in the alfuzosin trial. Possible reasons include the short treatment duration (≤ 12 weeks) and/or inclusion of refractory patients with previous exposure to alpha-blockers.

7.2.2.2 Antibiotic Therapy

Empirical antibiotic therapy is widely used because some patients have improved with antimicrobial therapy.

To date there are only three randomized controlled trials which assessed ciprofloxacin [28], levofloxacin [29], and tetracycline hydrochloride [30] vs. placebo in CP/CPPS patients. Although symptom improvement was observed, these studies failed to show a statistically significant improvement in NIH-CPSI total score from baseline to 6 weeks in a CP/CPPS population. More promising results were observed in a comparison of tetracycline hydrochloride vs. placebo, with significant differences in NIH-CPSI scores and bacterial eradication rates; however, patient numbers were small ($n = 48$) [30].

Combination therapy of antibiotics with *α-blockers* has shown even better outcomes in network meta-analysis. Despite significant improvement in symptom scores, antibiotic therapy did not lead to statistically significant higher response rates [31]. In addition, sample sizes of the studies were relatively small, and treatment effects were only modest and most of the time below clinical significance. It may be speculated that patients profiting from treatment have had some unrecognized uropathogens. If antibiotics are used, other therapeutic options should be offered after one unsuccessful course of a quinolone or tetracycline antibiotic over 2 weeks.

7.2.2.3 Pain Pharmacotherapies

Anti-inflammatory agents are considered the second line of pharmacotherapy for pain symptoms, along with α-adrenergic receptor antagonists (α-blockers) for urinary symptoms [32]. A 2009 randomized control trial evaluated celecoxib in CP/CPPS patients, with a statistically significant decrease in NIH-CPSI total ($p < 0.015$), pain ($p < 0.006$), and QoL ($p < 0.032$) scores after 2, 4, and 6 weeks; however, the effects were limited to the short duration of therapy [33].

Furthermore, two recent meta-analyses on anti-inflammatory therapy show mixed conclusions; one reported that NSAIDs were 80 % more likely to achieve a favorable response than placebo ($n=190$, relative risk [RR]: 1.8; 95 % confidence interval [CI]: 1.2–2.6), based on the combination of three trials evaluating rofecoxib, celecoxib, and a corticosteroid [26]. The second analysis, based on only the rofecoxib and celecoxib trials, concluded that no significant differences in efficacy could be ascertained for NSAIDs vs. placebo [27]. Overall, a moderate treatment effect has been shown for anti-inflammatory drugs, but larger studies are needed for confirmation, and long-term side effects have to be taken into account.

Opioids produce modest pain relief in some patients with refractory PPS, although there are limited data on the long-term efficacy of opioids in non-cancer pain. Opioid treatment carries the risk of side effects, reduced QoL, addiction, opioid tolerance, and opioid-induced hyperalgesia [34]. Urologists should use opioids for PPS only in collaboration with pain clinics and together with other treatments.

A randomized control trial evaluated pregabalin ($n=218$) vs. placebo ($n=106$) in the CP/CPPS population. Compared with the placebo group, patients in the pregabalin arm experienced reductions in the NIH-CPSI total score and subscores ($p<0.05$). However, pregabalin therapy for 6 weeks was not superior to placebo in the rate of a 6-point decrease in the NIH-CPSI total score [35].

7.2.2.4 5-Alpha-Reductase Inhibitors

The evidence base for the use of 5-alpha-reductase inhibitors in CP/CPPS is limited, with only three small ($n=41$–76) RCTs identified, which evaluated finasteride [36–38]. The first study showed that finasteride reduced pain and voiding symptoms vs. baseline; however, no statistically significant differences vs. a small and non-comparable control group were observed, which was likely due to lack of power. The second study compared finasteride with *Serenoa repens* (saw palmetto) and showed that patients treated with finasteride had a significant and enduring improvement (1-year trial duration) in NIH-CPSI total and pain domains, but not for urinary symptoms, when compared with baseline. However, the trial size ($n=64$) and lack of a placebo arm are significant warnings when interpreting the results of this study. A third study showed better outcomes, via measurements of subjective overall assessment and NIH-CPSI scores, for finasteride vs. placebo, but the results were not statistically significant.

The REDUCE study prospectively examined the effect of dutasteride vs. placebo in men with prostatitis-like pain (defined as NIH-CPSI pain subscore ≥ 5) and prostatitis-like syndrome (perineal or ejaculatory pain plus NIH-CPSI pain subscore ≥ 4) by evaluating NIH-CPSI scores at baseline and throughout the study (every 6 months for 4 years). NIH-CPSI total score decreased significantly at 48 months in the dutasteride group vs. placebo in men with prostatitis-like pain ($n=678$, $p<0.0001$) and with prostatitis-like syndrome ($n=427$, $p=0.03$). In addition, there were significantly more responders (defined as improvement of ≥ 4 units and ≥ 6 units in total CPSI score) with dutasteride vs. placebo for both prostatitis subgroup populations assessed. The REDUCE study was not primarily designed as a CP/CPPS treatment trial, but the significant reductions in NIH-CPSI scores compared with placebo in a relatively large patient cohort ($n = 1,105$) with prostatitis-like pain or syndrome suggest that use of 5-alpha-reductase inhibitors in older (aged ≥ 50 years) patients with PSA levels >2.5 ng/ml (for those aged 50–60 years) or >3.0 ng/ml (those aged >60 years) may be of clinical benefit [39].

7.2.2.5 Phytotherapy

Different studies assessed the effect of phytotherapy in CP/CPPS. Saw palmetto, pollen extracts, and pentosan polysulfate showed some improvement of pelvic pain in a few small studies [40]. Specifically, an adequately powered randomized placebo-controlled study of Cernilton showed clinically significant symptom improvement over a 12-week period in inflammatory PPS patients (NIH cat. IIIa) [41]. The effect was mainly based on an important effect on pain. Significant differences between another pollen extract (Prostat/Politt) and placebo were demonstrated in a small ($n = 60$) trial, but a validated tool for symptom scoring was not used [42]. Quercetin, a polyphenolic bioflavonoid with documented antioxidant and anti-inflammatory properties, improved NIH-CPSI scores significantly in a small RCT [43]. In contrast, treatment with saw palmetto, most commonly used for benign prostatic hyperplasia, did not improve symptoms over a 1-year period [36]. In a systematic review and meta-analysis, patients treated with phytotherapy were found to have significantly lower pain scores than those treated with placebo [26]. In addition, the overall response rate in network analysis was in favor of phytotherapy (RR: 1.6; 95 % CI: 1.1–1.6). A prospective, comparative trial provides additional evidence that phytotherapy offers symptom improvement in inflammatory CP/CPPS, with significant changes in symptoms from baseline observed for Profluss® (*Serenoa repens*, selenium, and lycopene) [44]. However, CP/CPPS patients treated with *Serenoa repens* reported no appreciable long-term improvement in NIH-CPSI scores in a 1-year comparative study vs. finasteride [36]. Recently the results of a randomized controlled phase III study assessing the safety and efficacy of pollen extract in association with vitamins in males with CP/CPPS were published. Participants were randomized to receive oral capsules of phytotherapeutic agent (two capsules every 24 h) or ibuprofen (600 mg, one tablet three times a day) for 4 weeks. At the follow-up examination (following 1 month of treatment), in the phytotherapeutic group, 31/41 patients (75.6 %) reported an improvement in quality of life, defined as a reduction of the NIH-CPSI total score by ≥ 25 %, compared with 19/46 (41.3 %) in the control group ($p = 0.002$) [45]. However, this topic has been discussed in detail based on published evidence in the next chapter of this book.

7.2.2.6 Pentosan Polysulfate

High-dose oral pentosan polysulfate (3×300 mg/day) is able to improve clinical global assessment and QoL significantly over placebo in men with PPS [46].

7.2.2.7 Diet, Sexual Habits, and Lifestyle

An Italian prospective randomized clinical trial showed that some potentially eliminable risk factors came from diet, sexual habits, and lifestyle and related to perineal trauma causing pelvic floor muscle tenderness. The majority of risk factors that were found to be associated with CPPS came from an abnormal diet and an irregular sexual life. Correction of these risk factors was important for the management of pelvic pain disease [47].

7.2.3 Physical Treatments

7.2.3.1 Extracorporeal Shockwave Therapy
A recent sham-controlled double-blind study ($n=30$) of perineal extracorporeal shockwave therapy four times weekly showed the potential benefit of this modality with significant improvement in pain, QoL, and voiding compared to the control group ($n=30$) over 12 weeks [48]. This procedure was performed without anesthesia or any noted significant side effects. This study showed for the first time encouraging results for a potentially promising and reliable new therapy for CP/CPPS.

7.2.3.2 Electromagnetic Therapy
In a small, sham-controlled, double-blind study, 4 weeks electromagnetic therapy showed a significant, sustained clinical improvement of symptomatology over a 1-year period [49].

7.2.3.3 Microwave Thermotherapy
Significant symptomatic improvement has been reported in uncontrolled studies of heat therapy, for example, based on the transrectal and transurethral thermotherapy [50, 51].

7.2.3.4 Electroacupuncture
In a small three-arm randomized trial, electroacupuncture was superior to sham treatment and advice and exercise alone [52]. In a recent prospective case series of 6 weeks of weekly electroacupuncture of 97 patients with PPS, 92 % showed significant improvement in total NIH-CPSI score.

7.2.3.5 Posterior Tibial Nerve Stimulation
One sham-controlled medium-sized study ($n=89$) demonstrated significant improvement in total NIH-CPSI score and visual analog scale for pain [53].

7.2.3.6 Myofascial Physical Therapy
A randomized feasibility trial of myofascial physical therapy including PPS ($n=21$) and patients with BPS showed a clinical benefit compared to global therapeutic massage [54]. In the PPS group alone, there was no difference in the effect between the two treatment arms.

7.2.3.7 Psychological Treatment
Even if a strong psychobiological component can be detected in some patients with long-standing CP/CPPS, the evidence for psychological treatment is still lacking. Only few data coming from uncontrolled trials have shown a weak evidence for improvement of pain and QoL, but not for urinary symptoms.

References

1. De la Rosette JJ et al (1993) Diagnosis and treatment of 409 patients with prostatitis syndromes. Urology 41(4):301–307
2. Tripp DA et al (2006) Catastrophizing and pain-contingent rest predict patient adjustment in men with chronic prostatitis/chronic pelvic pain syndrome. J Pain 7(10):697–708
3. Marszalek M et al (2007) Symptoms suggestive of chronic pelvic pain syndrome in an urban population: prevalence and associations with lower urinary tract symptoms and erectile function. J Urol 177(5):1815–1819
4. Walz J et al (2007) Impact of chronic prostatitis-like symptoms on the quality of life in a large group of men. BJU Int 100(6):1307–1311
5. Nickel JC (1998) Prostatitis: myths and realities. Urology 51(3):362–366
6. Barry MJ et al (2008) Overlap of different urological symptom complexes in a racially and ethnically diverse, community-based population of men and women. BJU Int 101(1):45–51
7. Roberts RO et al (2004) Low agreement between previous physician diagnosed prostatitis and national institutes of health chronic prostatitis symptom index pain measures. J Urol 171(1):279–283
8. Krieger JN et al (2008) Epidemiology of prostatitis. Int J Antimicrob Agents 31(Suppl 1): S85–S90
9. Mehik A et al (2000) Epidemiology of prostatitis in Finnish men: a population-based cross-sectional study. BJU Int 86(4):443–448
10. Engeler DS, Baranowski AP, Dinis-Oliveira P, Elneil S, Hughes J, Messelink EJ, van Ophoven A, Williams AC, European Association of Urology (2013) The 2013 EAU guidelines on chronic pelvic pain: is management of chronic pelvic pain a habit, a philosophy, or a science? 10 years of development. Eur Urol 64(3):431–439
11. Shoskes DA, Nickel JC, Dolinga R et al (2009) Clinical phenotyping of patients with chronic prostatitis/chronic pelvic pain syndrome and correlation with symptom severity. Urology 73:538–542, discussion 542–3
12. Shoskes DA, Nickel JC, Rackley RR et al (2009) Clinical phenotyping in chronic prostatitis/chronic pelvic pain syndrome and interstitial cystitis: a management strategy for urologic chronic pelvic pain syndromes. Prostate Cancer Prostatic Dis 12:177–183
13. Magri V, Wagenlehner F et al (2010) Use of the UPOINT chronic prostatitis/chronic pelvic pain syndrome classification in European patient cohorts: sexual function domain improves correlations. J Urol 184(6):2339–2345
14. Davis SN, Binik YM, Amsel R, Carrier S (2013) Is a sexual dysfunction domain important for quality of life in men with urological chronic pelvic pain syndrome? Signs "UPOINT" to yes. J Urol 189(1):146–151
15. Landis JR, Williams DA, Lucia MS et al (2014) The MAPP research network: design, patient characterization and operations. BMC Urol 14:58
16. Shoskes DA et al (2010) Phenotypically directed multimodal therapy for chronic prostatitis/chronic pelvic pain syndrome: a prospective study using UPOINT. Urology 75(6):1249–1253
17. Chen Y, Wu X, Liu J, Tang W, Zhao T, Zhang J (2011) Effects of a 6-month course of tamsulosin for chronic prostatitis/chronic pelvic pain syndrome: a multicenter, randomized trial. World J Urol 29:381–385
18. Nickel JC, Narayan P, McKay J, Doyle C (2004) Treatment of chronic prostatitis/chronic pelvic pain syndrome with tamsulosin: a randomized double blind trial. J Urol 171:1594–1597
19. Mehik A, Alas P, Nickel JC, Sarpola A, Helstrom PJ (2003) Alfuzosin treatment for chronic prostatitis/chronic pelvic pain syndrome: a prospective, randomized, double-blind, placebo-controlled, pilot study. Urology 62:425–429
20. Nickel JC, Krieger JN, McNaughton-Collins M et al (2008) Alfuzosin and symptoms of chronic prostatitis-chronic pelvic pain syndrome. N Engl J Med 18:2663–2673
21. Evliyaoglu Y, Burgut R (2002) Lower urinary tract symptoms, pain and quality of life assessment in chronic non-bacterial prostatitis patients treated with alpha-blocking agent doxazosin; versus placebo. Int Urol Nephrol 34:351–356

22. Tugcu V, Tasci AI, Fazlioglu A et al (2007) A placebo-controlled comparison of the efficiency of triple- and monotherapy in category III B chronic pelvic pain syndrome (CPPS). Eur Urol 51:1113–1117, discussion 8
23. Cheah PY, Liong ML, Yuen KH et al (2004) Initial, long-term, and durable responses to terazosin, placebo, or other therapies for chronic prostatitis/chronic pelvic pain syndrome. Urology 64:881–886
24. Gul O, Eroglu M, Ozok U (2001) Use of terazosine in patients with chronic pelvic pain syndrome and evaluation by prostatitis symptom score index. Int Urol Nephrol 32:433–436
25. Nickel JC, O'Leary MP, Lepor H et al (2011) Silodosin for men with chronic prostatitis/chronic pelvic pain syndrome: results of a phase II multicenter, double-blind, placebo controlled study. J Urol 186:125–131
26. Anothaisintawee T, Attia J, Nickel JC et al (2011) Management of chronic prostatitis/chronic pelvic pain syndrome: a systematic review and network meta-analysis. JAMA 305:78–86
27. Cohen JM, Fagin AP, Hariton E et al (2012) Therapeutic intervention for chronic prostatitis/chronic pelvic pain syndrome (CP/CPPS): a systematic review and meta-analysis. PLoS One 7:e41941
28. Alexander RB, Propert KJ, Schaeffer AJ et al (2004) Ciprofloxacin or tamsulosin in men with chronic prostatitis/chronic pelvic pain syndrome: a randomized, double-blind trial. Ann Intern Med 141:581–589
29. Nickel JC, Downey J, Clark J et al (2003) Levofloxacin for chronic prostatitis/chronic pelvic pain syndrome in men: a randomized placebo-controlled multicenter trial. Urology 62:614–617
30. Zhou Z, Hong L, Shen X et al (2008) Detection of nanobacteria infection in type III prostatitis. Urology 71:1091–1095
31. Thakkinstian A et al (2012) Alpha-blockers, antibiotics and anti-inflammatories have a role in the management of chronic prostatitis/chronic pelvic pain syndrome. BJU Int 110(7):1014–1022
32. Murphy AB, Macejko A, Taylor A, Nadler RB (2009) Chronic prostatitis: management strategies. Drugs 69:71–84
33. Zhao WP, Zhang ZG, Li XD et al (2009) Celecoxib reduces symptoms in men with difficult chronic pelvic pain syndrome (Category IIIA). Braz J Med Biol Res 42:963–967
34. Nickel JC (2006) Opioids for chronic prostatitis and interstitial cystitis: lessons learned from the 11th World Congress on Pain. Urology 68(4):697–701
35. Pontari MA, Krieger JN, Litwin MS et al (2010) Pregabalin for the treatment of men with chronic prostatitis/chronic pelvic pain syndrome: a randomized controlled trial. Arch Intern Med 170:1586–1593
36. Kaplan SA, Volpe MA, Te AE (2004) A prospective, 1-year trial using saw palmetto versus finasteride in the treatment of category III prostatitis/chronic pelvic pain syndrome. J Urol 171:284–288
37. Leskinen M, Lukkarinen O, Marttila T (1999) Effects of finasteride in patients with inflammatory chronic pelvic pain syndrome: a double-blind, placebo-controlled, pilot study. Urology 53:502–505
38. Nickel JC, Downey J, Pontari MA, Shoskes DA, Zeitlin SI (2004) A randomized placebo-controlled multicentre study to evaluate the safety and efficacy of finasteride for male chronic pelvic pain syndrome (category IIIA chronic nonbacterial prostatitis). BJU Int 93:991–995
39. Nickel JC et al (2011) Dutasteride reduces prostatitis symptoms compared with placebo in men enrolled in the REDUCE study. J Urol 186(4):1313–1318
40. Schaeffer AJ (2006) Clinical practice. Chronic prostatitis and the chronic pelvic pain syndrome. N Engl J Med 355:1690–1698
41. Wagenlehner FM et al (2009) A pollen extract (Cernilton) in patients with inflammatory chronic prostatitis-chronic pelvic pain syndrome: a multicentre, randomised, prospective, double-blind, placebo-controlled phase 3 study. Eur Urol 56(3):544–551

42. Elist J (2006) Effects of pollen extract preparation Prostat/Poltit on lower urinary tract symptoms in patients with chronic nonbacterial prostatitis/chronic pelvic pain syndrome: a randomized, double-blind, placebo-controlled study. Urology 67:60–63

43. Shoskes DA et al (1999) Quercetin in men with category III chronic prostatitis: a preliminary prospective, double-blind, placebo-controlled trial. Urology 54(6):960–963

44. Morgia G, Mucciardi G, Gali A et al (2010) Treatment of chronic prostatitis/chronic pelvic pain syndrome category IIIA with Serenoa repens plus selenium and lycopene (Profluss) versus S. repens alone: an Italian randomized multicenter-controlled study. Urol Int 84:400–406

45. Cai T, Wagenlehner FM, Luciani LG et al (2014) Pollen extract in association with vitamins provides early pain relief in patients affected by chronic prostatitis/chronic pelvic pain syndrome. Exp Ther Med 8(4):1032–1038

46. Nickel JC et al (2005) Pentosan polysulfate sodium therapy for men with chronic pelvic pain syndrome: a multicenter, randomized, placebo controlled study. J Urol 173(4):1252–1255

47. Gallo L (2014) Effectiveness of diet, sexual habits and lifestyle modifications on treatment of chronic pelvic pain syndrome. Prostate Cancer Prostatic Dis 17:238–245

48. Zimmermann R et al (2009) Extracorporeal shock wave therapy for the treatment of chronic pelvic pain syndrome in males: a randomised, double-blind, placebo-controlled study. Eur Urol 56(3):418–424

49. Rowe E et al (2005) A prospective, randomized, placebo controlled, double-blind study of pelvic electromagnetic therapy for the treatment of chronic pelvic pain syndrome with 1 year of followup. J Urol 173(6):2044–2047

50. Kastner C et al (2004) Cooled transurethral microwave thermotherapy for intractable chronic prostatitis–results of a pilot study after 1 year. Urology 64(6):1149–1154

51. Montorsi F et al (1993) Is there a role for transrectal microwave hyperthermia of the prostate in the treatment of abacterial prostatitis and prostatodynia? Prostate 22(2):139–146

52. Lee SH et al (2009) Electroacupuncture relieves pain in men with chronic prostatitis/chronic pelvic pain syndrome: three-arm randomized trial. Urology 73(5):1036–1041

53. Kabay S et al (2009) Efficiency of posterior tibial nerve stimulation in category IIIB chronic prostatitis/chronic pelvic pain: a Sham-Controlled Comparative Study. Urol Int 83(1):33–38

54. Fitzgerald MP et al (2013) Randomized multicenter feasibility trial of myofascial physical therapy for the treatment of urological chronic pelvic pain syndromes. J Urol 189(1 Suppl):S75–S85

The Role of Phytotherapy in the Management of Prostatitis Patients

8

Zafer Tandogdu and Mete Cek

8.1 Introduction

From an etymological perspective, phytotherapy involves the use of plants (phuton) to cure or alleviate illnesses (therapy). Plants have been a part of medicine long before modern medicine was founded and is still so. Human history has accumulated sporadic knowledge on the use of plants in medicine. However, there are two major deficiencies that limit the use of such knowledge. These are (i) the lack of systematic description of methods in acquiring and using the products and (ii) the lack of empirical proof of harms and benefits and . Luckily, modern medicine scientists have been a "good listener of the elderly" and tried to make use of this knowledge.

Current modern medicine applies the scientific methods in order to identify the safety, efficacy, and effectiveness of phytotherapeutics. Here, the difference between standard pharmacology and phytotherapeutics needs to be emphasized. *Standard pharmacology* identifies an active component to be used as a therapeutic. On the other hand, *phytotherapy* tries to identify and replicate the complex structure of a plant product as a potential therapeutic agent. In this chapter, we will not be referring to products that lack empirical data, which are accepted to be a part of complementary alternative medicine (CAM). For this purpose, a systematic review was carried out to identify randomized clinical trials (RCTs) and prospective cohort studies. Methodology for all studies was also appraised.

Chronic prostatitis/chronic pelvic pain syndrome (CP/CPPS) pathophysiology, clinical impact, and treatment options such as anti-inflammatories, alpha-blockers,

Z. Tandogdu (✉)
Urology working group within the NICR and the GHealth economics group in The IHS,
Northern Institute for Cancer Research Newcastle University – Institute for Health
and Society Newcastle University, Newcastle upon Tyne, UK
e-mail: drzafer@gmail.com

M. Cek
Department of Urology, Trakya Medical School, Edirne, Turkey

© Springer International Publishing Switzerland 2016
T. Cai, T.E. Bjerklund Johansen (eds.), *Prostatitis and Its Management: Concepts and Recommendations for Clinical Practice*, DOI 10.1007/978-3-319-25175-2_8

antimicrobials, etc. have been extensively discussed in other chapters of this book. Here, the phytotherapeutics that will be discussed are as follows: quercetin [1], pollen extracts (Cernilton) [2, 3], and saw palmetto (*Serenoa repens*) [4].

8.2   Clinical Evidence Used

Clinical evidence of phytotherapy applied in chronic prostatitis is limited with four studies. The study population in all studies was similar with NIH class III patients studied. However, prior to study, registration treatments received by patients was clear in only one study [3]. All of these studies were RCTs, but only one was methodologically robust [3].

8.3   Quercetin

Quercetin is a flavonoid and is abundant in apples, wine, and onions. Other sources of quercetin are berries, tea, pepper, radish, dill, and coriander. In vitro studies have shown its antioxidant [5], anti-inflammatory [6], and neuroprotective effects [7]. The potential therapeutic actions of quercetin are still to be proven with in vivo studies. The safe oral dose is 1,000 mg/day and up to 60 % of this is absorbed [8]. The absorbed amount is thought to be influenced by accompanied dietary intake [9]. Nevertheless, these rates are thought to be sufficient for quercetin to reveal its effects.

The clinical effects of quercetin in chronic prostatitis has been studied by Shoskes et al. [1]. Patients in this study were randomized to receive either quercetin 500 mg orally twice a day (*n*: 15) or placebo (*n*: 15) for 4 weeks. Both symptom scores and white blood cells seen in expressed prostatic secretion significantly improved in patients receiving quercetin compared to placebo (Table 8.1). These results need to be approached with caution as there are some methodological flaws such as low sample size and unclear exclusion criteria.

Table 8.1 Summary of RCTs conducted for phytotherapeutics in CP/CPPS

		Quercetin [1]		Pollen extract		Saw palmetto	
		Intervention	Placebo	Intervention	Placebo	Intervention	Finasteride
NIH-CPSI total score	Baseline	21 ± 1.8	20.2 ± 1.1	19.18	20.31	24.7 ± 5.1	23.9 ± 5.7
	After intervention	13 ± 1.7	18.8 ± 1.9	11.72	14.94	20	20
IPSS		NA	NA	−2.29 ± 0.44	−1.5 ± 0.44	−0.8	−0.5
Expressed prostatic secretion white blood cell count	Baseline	16.9 ± 5.1/hpf	13.1 ± 4.4/hpf	−5/hpf	−3/hpf	NR	
	After intervention	2.9 ± 1.8/hpf	8.3 ± 4.6/hpf				

hpf high-power field, *NR* not reported

8.4   Pollen Extract

The most common pollen extract substances are Cernitin GBX and Cernitin T60. The proposed mechanisms of action are as follows: anti-inflammatory [10], smooth muscle relaxation [11, 12], interference with prostatic androgen metabolism [13], and inhibition of prostatic stromal proliferation [14]. Prospective non-comparative studies have shown that pollen extracts may have benefits in patients with CP/CPPS. A recent RCT has shown that compared to placebo, Cernitin GBX + Cernitin T60 provides significant improvement in NIH-CPSI scores [3]. In this study, two capsules of 60 mg Cernitin T60 and 3 mg Cernitin GBX were administered three times a day for 12 weeks. The accompanying urethral stricture and bladder neck sclerosis are associated with less favorable outcomes [2]. Finally, Cai et al., by using a phase III RCT, showed that a complex with pollen extract in association with vitamins significantly improved total symptoms, pain, and quality of life compared with ibuprofen in patients with CP/CPPS, without severe side effects [15].

8.5   Saw Palmetto

Saw palmetto is a palmlike tree that has fruits (berries) rich in fatty acids and phytosterols. The extract of the berries is very popular as an alternative treatment for benign prostate hyperplasia (BPH). Although the mechanism of action of saw palmetto is not clear, it is thought that it has anti-inflammatory, antiandrogenic, and proapoptotic effects. Despite the popularity of saw palmetto among patients with BPH, an RCT published in 2011 and a Cochrane review published in 2009 have shown that it does not improve lower urinary tract symptoms in patients with BPH [16, 17].

In the only RCT conducted in patients with CP/CPPS, saw palmetto (325 mg per day) was compared with finasteride (5 mg per day) [4]. The improvement in NIH-CPSI total score and subdomains of pain was similar with both saw palmetto and finasteride. However, with finasteride, the treatment effect was seen to continue up to 12 months, while with saw palmetto, it deteriorated after the 3rd month. Currently, there are no placebo-controlled studies for saw palmetto. Nevertheless, with the RCT conducted, there seems to be benefit for patients and further studies may be warranted.

8.6   Comparison of Agents

The three best-studied phytotherapeutics in CP/CPPS, as mentioned above, are quercetin, pollen extracts, and saw palmetto. Among these, the methodologically most robust and satisfying study with the lowest risk of bias was done for pollen extracts by Wagenlehner et al. [3]. The results obtained from these studies have been summarized in Table 8.1. A similar improvement in NIH-CPSI score can be seen with all substances. The duration of improvement in symptoms for saw palmetto did not go beyond 3 months, while for pollen extracts, it was not measured after 3 months and with quercetin, it is not clear. A similar improvement in IPSS scores was seen with pollen extracts and saw palmetto. Finally, a decrease in WBC count in expressed prostatic secretion with quercetin and pollen extract was reported. Well safety and tolerability levels were reported for all substances.

Acknowledgments I would like to thank Prof. Truls Erik Bjerklund Johansen who has been a great mentor for me and supported me in this work as in many others. I also appreciate the hard work of Kezban Mirillo who assisted me in gathering the literature.

In conclusion, amongst phytotherapeutics Pollen extracts have the most convincing evidence for use in patients with CP/CPPS. Further studies for Quercetin and Saw palmetto are warranted as they have already proven to have benefits.

References

1. Shoskes DA et al (1999) Quercetin in men with category III chronic prostatitis: a preliminary prospective, double-blind, placebo-controlled trial. Urology 54(6):960–963
2. Rugendorff EW et al (1993) Results of treatment with pollen extract (Cernilton N) in chronic prostatitis and prostatodynia. Br J Urol 71(4):433–438
3. Wagenlehner FM et al (2009) A pollen extract (Cernilton) in patients with inflammatory chronic prostatitis-chronic pelvic pain syndrome: a multicentre, randomised, prospective, double-blind, placebo-controlled phase 3 study. Eur Urol 56(3):544–551
4. Kaplan SA, Volpe MA, Te AE (2004) A prospective, 1-year trial using saw palmetto versus finasteride in the treatment of category III prostatitis/chronic pelvic pain syndrome. J Urol 171(1):284–288
5. Min K, Ebeler SE (2009) Quercetin inhibits hydrogen peroxide-induced DNA damage and enhances DNA repair in Caco-2 cells. Food Chem Toxicol 47(11):2716–2722
6. Comalada M et al (2005) In vivo quercitrin anti-inflammatory effect involves release of quercetin, which inhibits inflammation through down-regulation of the NF-kappaB pathway. Eur J Immunol 35(2):584–592
7. Pandey AK et al (2012) Quercetin in hypoxia-induced oxidative stress: novel target for neuro-protection. Int Rev Neurobiol 102:107–146
8. Harwood M et al (2007) A critical review of the data related to the safety of quercetin and lack of evidence of in vivo toxicity, including lack of genotoxic/carcinogenic properties. Food Chem Toxicol 45(11):2179–2205
9. Cermak R, Landgraf S, Wolffram S (2003) The bioavailability of quercetin in pigs depends on the glycoside moiety and on dietary factors. J Nutr 133(9):2802–2807
10. Asakawa K et al (2001) Effects of cernitin pollen-extract (Cernilton) on inflammatory cytokines in sex-hormone-induced nonbacterial prostatitis rats. Hinyokika Kiyo 47(7):459–465
11. Habib FK et al (1990) In vitro evaluation of the pollen extract, cernitin T-60, in the regulation of prostate cell growth. Br J Urol 66(4):393–397
12. Kimura M et al (1986) Micturition activity of pollen extract: contractile effects on bladder and inhibitory effects on urethral smooth muscle of mouse and pig. Planta Med 2:148–151
13. Talpur N et al (2003) Comparison of Saw Palmetto (extract and whole berry) and Cernitin on prostate growth in rats. Mol Cell Biochem 250(1–2):21–26

14. Kamijo T, Sato S, Kitamura T (2001) Effect of cernitin pollen-extract on experimental nonbacterial prostatitis in rats. Prostate 49(2):122–131
15. Cai T, Wagenlehner FM, Luciani LG, Tiscione D, Malossini G, Verze P, Mirone V, Bartoletti R (2014) Pollen extract in association with vitamins provides early pain relief in patients affected by chronic prostatitis/chronic pelvic pain syndrome. Exp Ther Med 8(4):1032–1038
16. Barry MJ et al (2011) Effect of increasing doses of saw palmetto extract on lower urinary tract symptoms: a randomized trial. JAMA 306(12):1344–1351
17. Tacklind J et al (2012) Serenoa repens for benign prostatic hyperplasia. Cochrane Database Syst Rev (12):CD001423

Management of Infective Complications Following Prostate Biopsy

9

Truls E. Bjerklund Johansen, Catherine E.P. Pereira, and Vladimir Mouraviev

9.1 The Size of the Problem

9.1.1 Prevalence of Prostate Biopsies

An estimated one million sets of prostate biopsies are taken annually both in the USA and in the EU [1]. Approximately 30 % of patients have undergone at least one previous set of prostate biopsies [2].

9.1.2 Incidence of Infective Complications

In the early days of prostate biopsies before the widespread use of antibiotic prophylaxis, rates of urinary tract infection of over 60 % were reported following transrecal prostate biopsies [3]. There are several studies looking into the current rates of complications after prostate biopsies. These describe incidence rates for infective complications of roughly 5 % and similar rates for hospital readmissions. The huge number of biopsies carried out annually means that 100,000 men in the USA and the EU develop an infection as a result of prostate biopsy each year (5 % of two million). The risk of infection is three times higher in patients undergoing repeat biopsy [4, 5].

T.E.B. Johansen (✉)
Department of Urology, Oslo University Hospital, Oslo, Norway

Institute of Clinical Medicine, University of Aarhus, Aarhus, Denmark
e-mail: tebj@medisin.uio.no

C.E.P. Pereira
Department of Urology, Oslo University Hospital, Oslo, Norway

V. Mouraviev
Global Robotics Institute, Florida Hospital Celebration Health,
Celebration, Kissimmee, FL, USA

© Springer International Publishing Switzerland 2016
T. Cai, T.E. Bjerklund Johansen (eds.), *Prostatitis and Its Management: Concepts and Recommendations for Clinical Practice*, DOI 10.1007/978-3-319-25175-2_9

67

9.1.3 Type of Infections

About 4 % of patients experience febrile infective complications following prostate biopsy, but data describing the types of infections that can occur are not very reliable. Acute bacterial prostatitis and urosepsis are the most likely immediate infective complications. Urosepsis occurs less commonly, but is more severe. It is defined as evidence of urogenital tract infection plus the presence of at least two of the SIRS criteria [6, 7]. The most severe form of urosepsis is septic shock (Table 9.1). A febrile urinary tract infection indicates pyelonephritis. Epididymitis usually needs several days to develop. Complications from septicemia may present themselves after several weeks.

Table 9.1 Clinical presentation of cystitis (CY), pyelonephritis (PN), and urosepsis (US) and grading of severity [6, 21]

Acronym	Clinical diagnosis	Clinical symptoms	Grade of severity
CY-1	Cystitis	Dysuria, frequency, urgency, suprapubic pain; sometimes unspecific symptoms	1
PN-2	Mild and moderate pyelonephritis	Fever, flank pain, CVA tenderness; sometimes unspecific symptoms (see Table 9.1) with or without symptoms of CY	2
PN-3	Severe pyelonephritis	As PN-2, but in addition nausea and vomiting with or without symptoms of CY	3
US-4	Urosepsis (simple)	(>2 SIRS criteria must be met for US-4 diagnosis) Temperature > 38 °C or < 36 °C Heart rate >90 beats min Respiratory rate >20 breaths/min or $PaCO_2$ <32 mmHg (<4.3kPa) WBC >12,000 cells/mm^3 or <4000 cells/mm^3 or $\geq$10 % immature (band) forms With or without symptoms of CY or PN	4
US-5	Severe urosepsis	As US-4, but in addition associated with organ dysfunction, hypoperfusion, or hypotension Hypoperfusion and perfusion abnormalities may include but are not limited to lactic acidosis, oliguria, or an acute alteration of mental status	5
US-6	Uroseptic shock	AS US-4 or US-5, but in addition with hypotension despite adequate fluid resuscitation along with the presence of perfusion abnormalities that may include, but are not limited to lactic acidosis, oliguria, or an acute alteration in mental status. Patients who are on inotropic or vasopressor agents may not be hypotensive at the time that perfusion abnormalities are measured	6

9.1.4   Mortality and Costs

SIRS and urosepsis are associated with significant mortality rates, rising from as high as 7 % for SIRS to 46 % for septic shock [8]. Mortality following prostate biopsies is rare and most deaths are associated with septic shock. A 30-day mortality rate of 0.1–0.2 % has been reported after prostate biopsies [9, 10]. Figures are uncertain, but a mortality rate of 0.2 % translates to 4000 men dying from prostate biopsies in the USA and EU every year.

The costs associated with readmissions were studied in the UK in 2013 and were estimated to 4260 £ per patient readmitted [11]. With an exchange rate of 1.352, the costs of readmissions after prostate biopsies for Europe only amount to 290 million Euros per year.

9.2   Indications for Prostate Biopsies

Prostate biopsy is a prerequisite for a histological diagnosis of prostate cancer which in turn is a prerequisite for curative treatment. A key consideration before carrying out a prostate biopsy is whether the benefit of diagnosis outweighs the potential side effects of the procedure. A prostate biopsy should not be performed unless the histological findings will be of benefit to the patient. Several scenarios should be considered.

9.2.1   Radical Treatment

If radical treatment is considered, biopsies should only be performed if the patient meets the inclusion criteria for age and comorbidity. If these criteria are met, biopsies should be performed in a standardized manner where all regions of the prostate are biopsied, usually by means of 10–12 cores [6].

9.2.2   Focal Treatment

If focal treatment is considered, prostate biopsies have a double role, to *rule in* prostate cancer in the part of the prostate that will be treated and to *rule out* prostate cancer from the regions of the gland that is not going to be treated. Ruling out prostate cancer usually requires more biopsies than when the objective is to *rule in* before treatment. Ruling out biopsies is often done in a second procedure within few months of the primary biopsies. In such cases, a different antibiotic prophylaxis should be considered [12, 13].

9.2.3 Active Surveillance and Watchful Waiting

If radical treatment is postponed for a patient with low-grade prostate cancer, the patient will most likely come back for repeat biopsies to monitor the progress of the tumor. The increased risk of infective complications for repeat biopsies should be discussed with the patient before including him in a surveillance protocol.

9.2.4 Palliative Treatment

Sometimes patients present with clear evidence of metastatic or locally advanced prostate cancer such as elevated PSA, metastases on imaging, and characteristic findings on DRE. Often these patients are older, have a catheter and a preexisting bacteriuria, and thus are at increased risk of infection after prostate biopsies. In such patients, starting reversible hormone treatment without histological confirmation of diagnosis may be justified.

9.3 Technical Aspects of Prostate Biopsies and the Risk of Infective Complications

Tissue specimens for diagnosing prostate cancer may be obtained in different ways. Biopsy techniques differ in terms of approach and guidance. The detection rate of cancer and the risk of infection are major considerations when deciding which technique to use.

9.3.1 The Good Old Days

Before the era of PSA, men with prostate cancer presented with voiding problems and underwent transurethral resection with minimal risks of side effects. Diagnosis was based on histological examination of TURP (transurethral resection of the prostate) specimens. When patients came to discuss prostate cancer treatment, their voiding problems were solved and their potency was preserved.

Today patients present with elevated PSA, usually in the absence of voiding problems, to discuss if a biopsy shall be taken. Already at that time point we have to discuss if they are willing to sacrifice their potency and continence in the event that a biopsy reveals prostate cancer and radical prostatectomy is recommended.

9.3.2 Transrectal Approach

The transrectal approach is the most commonly used. The biopsies are either taken through a side-fire channel at an angle of 22° to the probe, or through an end-fire channel parallel to the probe. Using a side-fire probe, the biopsies are mainly taken from the posterior part of the prostate, and sampling the apical region is difficult. An end-fire probe enables easier sampling of the anterior part and the apical region.

In both methods, the biopsy needle traverses the same channel in the probe and passes through the rectal wall each time a core is taken. Usually, the same biopsy needle is used for all cores.

9.3.3 Perineal Approach

Perineal biopsies are also taken by way of a transrectal ultrasound probe, but the needle is steered through the holes in a metal template which is mounted on a stepper and also carries the ultrasound probe (Fig. 9.1). Transperineal biopsies are technically demanding because the needle has to travel a longer distance and may more easily change its course inside the prostate. However, the skin can be disinfected and the needle does not have to pierce the rectal wall so the procedure is less contaminated than the transrectal approach.

New equipment is available which makes use of a single channel through the skin and the pelvic floor for all biopsies. Due to the reduced contamination, the risk of infective complications is also lower [14]. However, transperineal biopsies require sedation or general anesthesia, the setup is more resource demanding and other side effects may be significant [15].

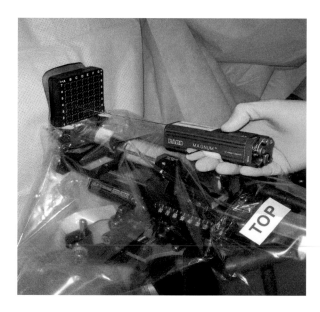

Fig. 9.1 Setup for transperineal prostate biopsies showing the ultrasound probe in the rectum: the steel template and the biopsy needle passing through a hole in the template (Courtesy of W. Barzell, Florida)

9.3.4 Biopsy Guidance and Tracking

The most commonly used method of guidance is transrectal ultrasound. In patients that have been operated with amputation of the rectum, transperineal biopsies may be guided by a transabdominal probe. In conventional ultrasound-guided biopsies, the needle is usually removed immediately after a core has been taken.

With image-fusion systems and MRI-guided biopsies, the needle must remain inside the prostate while its position is being tracked either by scanning with 3D ultrasound or while new MR images are taken. Furthermore, image-fusion biopsies are more commonly used when anterior tumors are suspected. This means that the tip of the biopsy needle often travels all the way through the prostate and into the veins on the anterior surface of the gland. Image-fusion-guided biopsies are also often repeat biopsies. These factors may increase the risk of infective complications.

9.4 Patient Selection and How to Reduce the Need for Prostate Biopsies

A biomarker that could reduce the number of biopsies and improve detection of significant prostate cancer would be of great importance. However, with an autopsy prevalence for prostate cancer of more than 50 % in 60-year-old males, there is still a long way to go from the sensitivity of the tests currently available [16].

9.4.1 Digital Rectal Examination (DRE)

A meta-analysis of DRE estimated its sensitivity for detecting prostate cancer to be 59 % and its specificity 94 % [17]. This means that DRE cannot be used to rule out prostate cancer in a patient with elevated PSA.

9.4.2 Biomarkers

Most patients are referred to prostate biopsy because of elevated PSA on repeat examinations after excluding urinary tract infections and prostatitis. The sensitivity of PSA as judged by classical screening biopsies and a PSA cutoff of 4.0 ng/mL was 21 % for detecting any prostate cancer. This means that 79 % of tests are falsely negative, a fact that explains why patients with a persistently elevated PSA keep coming back for repeat biopsies [18]. The low sensitivity of PSA is a strong argument for better biomarkers. Long noncoding (lnc) RNAs like PCA3, ANRIL/P15AS, PCAT1, PCGM1, PTENP1, SChLAP1, and SPKY4-IT1 are appearing as the next generation of biomarkers expected to significantly improve early diagnosis, risk stratification, treatment monitoring, and even targeted treatment [19].

9.4.3 Imaging

During the last decade, we have witnessed rapid developments in the use of MRI for diagnosis and staging of prostate cancer. Initially, MRI findings were used as a targeting aid for cognitively guided TRUS (transrectal ultrasound guided) biopsies. This technique has now been replaced by image-fusion systems which enable the replacement of random biopsies with a few targeted biopsies and precise recording of biopsy sites (Fig. 9.2). MRI has improved T-staging and the planning of radical treatment.

In the recent few years, MRI has also been introduced to rule out prostate cancer. Although the negative predictive value of MRI in elite centers is high, there is not yet enough data to support the widespread use of MRI as a screening tool [6].

9.4.4 Reducing the Number of Cores

While MRI may not do away with the need for prostate biopsies altogether, it may reduce the number of cores taken per biopsy procedure by facilitating targeted prostate biopsies and reduce the need for repeat biopsies. Unfortunately, there is still no evidence that this will reduce the number of infective complications, but this is definitely an important research question. Before we can study this, we need better knowledge about the negative predictive value of MRI.

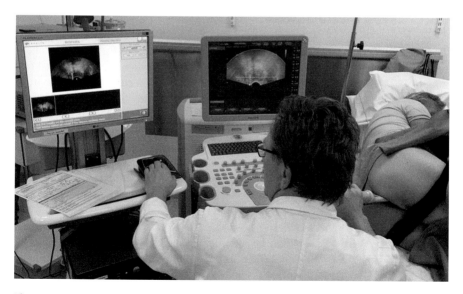

Fig. 9.2 Setup for image-fusion-guided prostate biopsies with the Koelis system. The urologist is simulating biopsy position on the Koelis computer with his left hand while positioning the 3-D sonotrode by means of his right hand. The screen to the right shows live ultrasound pictures (Courtesy of E. Baco, Norway)

9.4.5 Repeat Biopsy

Comparative studies are not available, but we know from observational studies that the risk of infective complications after repeat biopsies is approximately 15 % [4, 5]. Therefore, any measure that will reduce the need for repeat biopsies is important. Today patients who are coming in for repeat biopsies either have a rising PSA and negative screening biopsies or are in a surveillance program. It is expected that early MRI followed by targeted biopsies may reduce the need for repeat biopsies, particularly for patients who are shown to have anterior tumors. With better negative predictive value, MRI is also expected to reduce the need for repeat biopsies in surveillance programs.

9.4.6 Order of Screening Tools

The sequence of screening steps remains analysis of PSA followed by random biopsies. The best way to avoid infective complications is to avoid repeat biopsies. Better biomarkers and imaging techniques with better negative predictive values are important research areas.

9.5 Reducing the Impact of Patient-Related Risk Factors

9.5.1 Take a Careful History

The most important specific risk factor for the development of infective complications after prostate biopsy is antibiotic treatment or prophylaxis within the last few months [20]. Other risk factors that increase the chance of a contaminated environment are an indwelling catheter, a history of urinary tract infection or prostatitis, and travel to regions with a high prevalence of antibiotic resistance. Also important are comorbidities that reduce the immunocompetence of the patient such as diabetes, smoking, and a range of immunocompromising treatments. Disturbances in coagulation, for example, use of anticoagulants, are important for the risk of bleeding.

The ESIU/EAU (European Section for Infections in Urology/European Association of Urology) recently introduced the concept of phenotyping to better describe the different groups of risk factors for urogenital infections, the so-called ORENUC system (Table 9.2) [21]. The system has six main categories. Each category is referred to by a letter and all letters together give the name ORENUC. A history of UTI during the recent 6 months or asymptomatic bacteriuria are important category U risk factors, while having an indwelling catheter is a category C risk factor.

A careful history prior to prostate biopsy helps the clinician to tailor the prophylaxis to the patient and to identify risk factors that must be considered or eliminated in order to avoid complications.

Table 9.2 Host risk factors in urinary tract infections categorized according to the ORENUC system [6, 21]

Phenotype	Category of risk factor	Examples of risk factors
O	NO known risk factor	Otherwise healthy premenopausal women
R	Risk factors for Recurrent UTI, but no risk of more severe outcome	Sexual behavior (frequency, spermicide)
		Hormonal deficiency in postmenopause
		Secretor type of certain blood groups
		Well-controlled diabetes mellitus
E	Extra-urogenital risk factors with risk of more severe outcome	Prematurity, newborn
		Pregnancy
		Male gender
		Badly controlled diabetes mellitus
		Relevant immunosuppression (not well defined)
N	Nephropathic diseases with risk of more severe outcome	Relevant renal insufficiency (not well defined)
		Polycystic nephropathy
		Interstitial nephritis, e.g., due to analgesics
U	Urological risk factors with risk of more severe outcome, which can be resolved during therapy	Ureteral obstruction due to a ureteral stone
		Well-controlled neurogenic bladder disturbances
		Transient short-term external urinary catheter
		Asymptomatic bacteriuria
C	Permanent urinary Catheter and non-resolvable urological risk factors with risk of more severe outcome	Long-term external urinary catheter
		Non-resolvable urinary obstruction
		Badly controlled neurogenic bladder disturbances

9.5.2 Perform a Relevant Clinical Examination

The fact that some patients do not have rectum must not be overlooked. Before a patient is scheduled for prostate biopsy, it must be checked that a digital rectal examination (DRE) has been performed and that the anus is passable for a sonotrode. A urine culture should be taken if there is a history of urinary tract infection or prostatitis. Otherwise, a urine dipstick test is adequate. A rectal swab is recommended if there is a risk for fluoroquinolone-resistant or ESBL-producing bacteria.

The need for a thorough discussion about the indication for biopsy, the work-up necessary based on the clinical history, a clinical examination, and the performance of screening tests are arguments for not carrying out biopsies at the first visit. This also enables the patient to give fully informed consent for the biopsy procedure.

9.6   Reducing the Contamination Status of the Biopsy Procedure

9.6.1   The Local Microbiome

The diversity and the number of microorganisms in the rectum are well known. Pathogenic microorganisms may enter the body through natural orifices during travel and hospital stays and will soon colonize the rectum and the perineum. After exposure to ciprofloxacin, for example, during prophylaxis for a previous biopsy or treatment of a urinary tract infection, the risk of carrying ciprofloxacin-resistant bacteria in the rectum is about 50 % [12, 13].

Even in the absence of clinical signs of prostatitis, dormant microorganisms are present in the prostate in up to 90 % of males undergoing transurethral resection for benign prostatic obstruction [22]. With modern gene-sequencing techniques, we can demonstrate a world of microorganisms in the prostate below the detection capability of culture tests.

9.6.2   Contamination Categories of Prostate Biopsies

The risk of developing infective complications after surgical procedures depends on the local microbiome and the vitality of the tissue in the surgical field. Other important factors for assessment of the contamination of a surgical procedure are if a bodily tract is opened and there is spillage of its contents [23]. Contamination is graded into *Contamination categories* (Textbox 9.1). Large databases describe the infection rate in each category and confirm the validity of the classification principle [23, 24]. The ESIU recently worked out separate definitions for contamination categories in urology. Table 9.3 shows the categories and the corresponding risks of infective complications after prostate biopsy [6, 25].

> **Textbox 9.1. Classical Definitions of Surgical Field Contamination**
>   I. Clean
> II. Clean contaminated
> III. Contaminated
> IV. Dirty

9.6.3   Altering the Contamination Category

Transperineal biopsies have a lower contamination category than transrectal biopsies. Patient-related risk factors like bacteriuria will increase the contamination category. Performing biopsies in patients with indwelling transurethral catheters should be avoided when possible. If biopsy cannot be avoided, administration of antibiotics should be regarded as treatment, not prophylaxis.

Table 9.3 Biopsy routes, contamination categories, and risk of infection without prophylaxis in prostate biopsies [6, 25]

Biopsy route	Contamination category	Key criteria	Risk of infection (%)
	Clean		<5
Transperineal	Clean contaminated	Sterile urine	5–10
		No history UTI/UGI	
Transperineal	Contaminated	Sterile urine	10–15
		History of UTI/UGI	
Transrectal	Contaminated	Sterile urine	10–15
Transrectal	Dirty	Bacteriuria	15–40
		Urethral catheter	

UTI urinary tract infection, *UGI* urogenital infection (i.e., prostatitis)

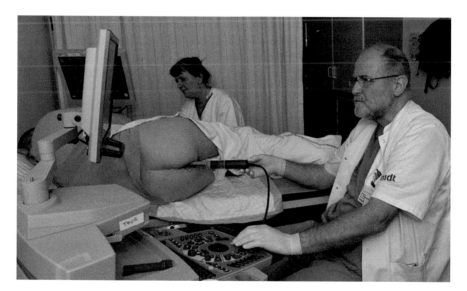

Fig. 9.3 Setup for conventional 3-D ultrasound-guided prostate biopsies. The urologist and the patient are in convenient positions. The patient watches the procedure on a separate screen and is continuously informed by the assistant. No local anesthetic is used (Courtesy of K. Pedersen, Denmark)

Transrectal biopsies are commonly carried out under local anesthesia. However, cyst-like accumulations of local anesthetic which are later repeatedly traversed by the biopsy needle may further increase the risk of infection. Informing the patient carefully about the procedure and even providing them with a separate ultrasound screen may reduce the need for local anesthesia (Fig. 9.3). Patients should lie as conveniently as possible, both for themselves and for the urologist. Most right-handed urologists prefer to have the patient in a left side-lying position. Transperineal biopsies are usually carried out under sedation or general anesthesia and local anesthesia is not routinely used.

9.6.4   Rectal Cleansing

Emptying the rectum with an enema makes insertion of the probe easier and improves visibility.

The effect of disinfection of the rectal mucosa has been evaluated for bisacodyl and povidone-iodine, respectively, with and without antibiotic prophylaxis. A significant decrease of infectious complications was found in a cohort where rectal preparation using bisacodyl was employed [26]. A clinically relevant, but not statistically significant, difference was found for povidone-iodine in a similar study [27]. Rectal cleansing is a simple means of reducing infection risk without increasing antibiotic resistance.

9.6.5   The Role of Hygienic Measures

Using the same needle for repeated biopsies through a contaminated field violates the principles for surgical hygiene. However, since the biopsy channel in the ultrasound probe cannot be disinfected during the procedure, using a new needle for each biopsy would not reduce contamination and would significantly increase costs.

The urologist should make sure that the cores are placed on a sterile backing and that the needle is protected as much as possible from contamination during the procedure. It is important that not only the urologist but also the assistant are properly trained and are familiar with hygienic principles.

9.7   Antibiotic Prophylaxis

9.7.1   General Considerations

Antibiotic prophylaxis is about delivering an antibiotic that is effective against the most likely pathogens, to a certain body region in a certain concentration during a certain period of time. Prevention of infection in an individual should not unnecessarily contribute to antibiotic resistance in common bacteria in the general patient population. The above considerations are about pharmacodynamics, pharmacokinetics, and collateral effects of antibiotics [28].

The concentration of an antibiotic in the prostate by the time of the biopsy is more important than its concentration in the blood. However, the exact concentration required in the prostate for effect is unknown and also depends on the MIC (minimal inhibitory concentration) of the pathogen. Of all evaluated antibiotic substance groups, fluoroquinolones and macrolides are best investigated and exhibit the highest serum – prostate secretion/tissue ratios [29–32]. Beta-lactam antibiotics such as piperacillin, cefpodoxime, meropenem, or doripenem reach concentrations in the prostate of only 10–20 % of plasma concentrations [32–34], while trimethoprim exhibits concentrations that, in one study, were higher than in serum [35].

Unfortunately, many broad-spectrum antibiotics promote the development of multiresistant pathogens such as extended-spectrum beta-lactamase (ESBL) producing Enterobacteriaceae, vancomycin-resistant *Enterococci* (VRE), fluoroquinolone-resistant *P. aeruginosa*, methicillin-resistant *Staphylococci* (MRSA), and growth of *C. difficile*. This phenomenon is called associated resistance and is an example of the collateral effects of antibiotics [36].

9.7.2 Recommended Prophylactic Regimens

Many antibiotics are suitable for perioperative antibacterial prophylaxis, e.g., fluoroquinolones, co-trimoxazole, second-generation cephalosporins, aminopenicillins plus a beta-lactamase inhibitor (BLI), and aminoglycosides. However, as a general rule, broad-spectrum antibiotics such as the fluoroquinolones, third-generation cephalosporins, and the carbapenem group should be used sparingly and reserved for treatment. This applies also to the use of vancomycin [6].

Fluoroquinolones are recommended as first-choice prophylaxis for prostate biopsies due to their favorable pharmacokinetic and pharmacodynamic properties and evidence of their effect from clinical studies. Alternative antibiotics include trimethoprim/sulfamethoxazole, cephalosporins, and (acyl)aminopenicillins/beta-lactamase inhibitors. There is no clinical evidence to support the addition of metronidazole.

A single dose of antibiotic is recommended in low-risk patients. A prolonged course can be considered in patients with risk factors [6].

9.7.3 When to Use Alternative Regimens

Alternative regimens should be considered when fluoroquinolone-resistant bacteria are detected in the rectal flora, after recent administration of fluoroquinolones, after recent travel to high-risk regions, and for repeat biopsies. The MIC value should be considered when choosing the concentration of fluoroquinolone-selective agar used to screen for rectal fluoroquinolone-resistant bacteria [37].

The prevalence of ESBL-producing bacteria is increasing and has reached 30 % in many countries. Since fluoroquinolones are not beta-lactam antibiotics, the presence of ESBL-producing bacteria is not an argument for an alternative prophylactic regimen. However, the presence of ESBL-producing bacteria is associated with more complications following biopsies, and the urologist should be prepared for the possibility that beta-lactam antibiotics may not be effective when infections occur.

Trimethoprim/sulfamethoxazole is not recommended for prophylaxis in regions where the general resistance rate is >20 %.

9.7.4   Local Protocols

There are considerable variations between countries when it comes to bacterial spectra and susceptibility to antibiotics. Antimicrobial resistance is usually higher in the Mediterranean region and in Asia as compared with Northern European countries [38]. The spread of multiresistance is a concern.

Knowledge about the local pathogen profile, the predominant pathogens causing infections after prostate biopsies, susceptibility, and virulence are each important for establishing local antibiotic guidelines. It is therefore recommended to establish a local multidisciplinary team of microbiologists, infectious disease specialists, and urologists to discuss surveillance programs and protocols for prophylaxis and empiric antibiotic treatment.

9.8   The Biopsy Procedure

9.8.1   Before the Procedure

Take a time-out and do a safety check:

- Is there a clear indication?
- Have you considered all contraindications and risk factors?
- Has the patient's urine and rectum been screened according to your protocol?
- Is the patient adequately prepared with enema and rectal cleansing?
- Has antibiotic prophylaxis been given at the right time?
- Is the patient fully informed and able to give an informed consent?

9.8.2   During the Procedure

Place the patient in a comfortable position. Demonstrate the sound of the biopsy gun to the patient. Wait until the local anesthesia is effective before taking biopsies. Inform the patient before each core is taken during the procedure. Make sure that all areas of interest are biopsied and try to avoid the need for repeat biopsy; check that all cores are correctly numbered and side oriented. Stretch the cores out before fixation and ink the tip if relevant. Check that the referral letter to the pathologist is readable and easily understood, also by your fellow urologists.

9.8.3   After the Procedure

Inform the patient about what has been done and tell him about the possible complications and what he should do if he experiences a complication: When to seek medical advice or treatment, who to contact, and what information to give. Give the patient written information about the procedure and the prophylaxis he received.

9.9   Diagnosing Infective Complications

9.9.1   Diagnosis and Severity Grading

Febrile infections occurring after prostate biopsies are most often urogenital or male accessory gland infections, urinary tract infections, and sepsis or septic foci in remote sites. Relevant urogenital infections (UGI) are prostatitis and epididymitis. A urinary tract infection is classified as cystitis (CY), pyelonephritis (PN), and urosepsis (US). The clinical presentation is always the most important prognostic criterion.

In acute prostatitis, the patient may have pelvic pain and urinary retention, and there is prostate tenderness on DRE. The clinical presentation of the three urinary tract entities and urosepsis is presented in Table 9.1. The ESIU has suggested to ascribe each of the clinical presentations a severity grade in Arabic letters (Table 9.1) [6, 21]. Urosepsis is always the most severe type of UTI and a PN is always more severe than a CY. According to ESIU/EAU definitions, a patient has a symptomatic urogenital infection (UTI) if:

- There are clinical symptoms indicative of urogenital infection
- Pathogens can be verified or suspected by culture, microscopy, dipstick, or PCR techniques
- Diagnosis of or prescription of an appropriate therapy for symptomatic urogenital infection is made/given by a physician upon clinical evaluation [21]

Febrile infections occurring within the first week after prostate biopsy are most often acute prostatitis or urosepsis. Infections that present later are most often epididymitis or complications of septicemia (Fig. 9.4). Systemic symptoms of acute prostatitis and urosepsis are similar and making a clinical diagnosis is sometimes difficult. PN can also present as a severe infection with systemic reactions like nausea and

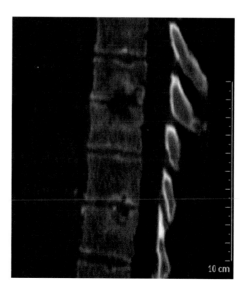

Fig. 9.4 CT scan showing septic spondylitis in a man who developed septicemia after prostate biopsies

vomiting. The three entities can be differentiated using the SIRS criteria. Sepsis is a sign of imminent physiological collapse and vital signs must be followed carefully. Patients with febrile infections after prostate biopsy should be hospitalized.

9.9.2 Specimens for Culture

Blood and urine cultures should be taken before initiation of empiric antibiotic therapy. Prostatic massage is contraindicated.

9.9.3 Imaging

Unless the patient responds rapidly to antibiotic treatment, imaging of the urinary tract and the prostate should be performed. The urinary tract is examined with CT urography and the prostate with transrectal ultrasound or MRI. The objective is to look for urinary retention on any level and a prostatic abscess.

9.10 Treatment of Infective Complications

When infective complications develop in patients who received antibiotic prophylaxis, the causative agent can be assumed resistant to this antibiotic. Therefore, as a rule, the prophylactic antibiotic should not be given for treatment. The most important infective complications are acute bacterial prostatitis, urosepsis, and pyelonephritis. All of these infections are hospital-acquired infections by definition. The goal for antibiotic therapy of hospital-acquired infections is not only to cure the patient but also to contain the spread of infection and prevent the emergence of resistant mutants. Although empiric therapy must be instigated immediately after microbiological sampling, the outcome of susceptibility testing can serve to narrow the antibiotic coverage.

9.10.1 Acute Bacterial Prostatitis

Parenteral administration of high doses of bactericidal antibiotics, such as broad-spectrum penicillin, a third-generation cephalosporin, or a fluoroquinolone should be administered. For initial therapy, any of these antibiotics may be combined with an aminoglycoside. After defeverescence and normalization of infection parameters, intravenous therapy can be replaced by oral therapy and continued for a total of 2–4 weeks [39].

A bladder catheter should be inserted in case of retention, but not as a routine measure. A prostatic abscess may be drained by transrectal puncture or transurethral de-roofing depending on the size and position of the abscess and the condition of the patient.

9.10.2 Urosepsis

The primary concern should be early, goal-directed therapy in order to maintain adequate circulation and oxygenation. According to the Surviving Sepsis Campaign [7], the critical values are as follows:

- Central venous pressure (CVP) of 8–12 mmHg
- Mean arterial pressure (MAP) of 65–90 mmHg
- Central venous oxygen (CVO_2) ≥ 70 %
- Hematocrit (HKT) >30 %
- Urine output >40 mL/h

Initial empirical antibiotic treatment should provide broad coverage. Treatment should be adapted as soon as culture results are available. The dosage of the antibiotics is of paramount importance in the sepsis syndrome and should generally be high, with the exception of patients in renal failure. Antimicrobials must be administered no later than 1 h after clinical diagnosis of sepsis.

The antibacterial treatment options include cephalosporins (group 3a/b), fluoroquinolones anti-*Pseudomonas* active acylaminopenicillins/BLI, and carbapenems. Any of these may be combined with an aminoglycoside. Treatment should be continued until 3–5 days after defeverescence or control/elimination of complicating factors [6].

Patients must be observed on a continuous basis and the urologist should consider repeatedly if the patient should be transferred to a high dependency unit or the intensive care department. If signs of organ dysfunction or refractory hypotension develop, the mortality rate can exceed 40 % [7]. If imaging reveals urinary retention or an abscess, proper drainage and source control are crucial.

9.10.3 Severe Pyelonephritis

This form of PN usually needs initial parenteral therapy and hospitalization. Antibiotic treatment can be started with an aminopenicillin/BL, oral cephalosporin (group 2 or 3a), or an anti-*Pseudomonas* active fluoroquinolone unless one has already been given as prophylaxis. Any of these may be combined with an aminoglycoside.

If there is no clinical improvement after 2–3 days, an acylaminopenicillin/BLI, cephalosporin (group 3b), or carbapenem can be given with or without an aminoglycoside. If *Candida* is cultured, fluconazole or amphotericin B should be given. Treatment should continue for at least 3–5 days beyond defeverescence, depending on the removal of risk factors [6]. PN can also present as a mild or moderate infection, which may be treated with oral antimicrobials in an outpatient setting.

9.11 Perspectives

Infective complications after prostate biopsies can be a significant threat to patients' health, and the benefit of diagnosing prostate cancer must always be considered against side effects before a biopsy is performed.

Due to the vast numbers of biopsies taken and the costs of readmission, infectious complications have become a significant public health problem. The increasing antibiotic resistance makes prophylaxis and treatment more difficult and adds to the severity of the situation.

The use of antibiotics and the infective complications after prostate biopsies should be surveyed prospectively in an international registry. Future research should be directed at the possibility of reducing the need for prostate biopsies and the contamination status of the biopsy procedure.

References

1. Loeb S, Carter HB, Berndt SI, Ricker W, Schaeffer EM (2011) Complications after prostate biopsy: data from SEER-Medicare. J Urol 186:1830–1834
2. Wagenlehner FM et al (2013) Infective complications after prostate biopsy: outcome of the global prevalence study of infections in urology (GPIU) 2010 and 2011, a prospective multinational multicentre prostate biopsy study. Eur Urol 63:521–527
3. Crawford ED, Haynes AL Jr, Story MW, Borden TA (1982) Prevention of urinary tract infection and sepsis following transrectal prostatic biopsy. J Urol 127(3):449–451
4. Ehdaie B, Vertosick E, Spaliviero M et al (2014) The impact of repeat biopsies on infectious complications in men with prostate cancer on active surveillance. J Urol 191:660–664
5. Birkebæk FT, Berg KD, Iversen P, Brasso K (2015) Poor association between the progression criteria in active surveillance and subsequent histopathological findings following radical prostatectomy. Scandinavian J Urol 49:1–6. doi:10.3109/21681805.2015.1040448
6. European Association of Urology. Individual guidelines.www.uroweb.org/guidelines (4.3.2015)
7. Dellinger RP et al (2012) Surviving sepsis campaign: international guidelines for management of severe sepsis and septic shock. Crit Care Med 41:580–637
8. Rangel-Frausto MS, Pittet D, Costigan M et al (1995) The natural history of the systemic inflammatory response syndrome (SIRS). A prospective study. JAMA 273(2):117–123
9. Nam RK et al (2010) Increasing hospital admission rates for urological complications after transrectal ultrasound guided prostate biopsy. J Urol 183:963–968
10. Carmignani L et al (2012) Bacterial sepsis following prostatic biopsy. Int Urol Nephrol 44:1055–1063
11. Batura D, Gopal Rao G (2013) The national burden of infections after prostate biopsy in England and Wales: a wake-up call for better prevention. J Antimicrob Chemother 68:247–249
12. Wagenlehner F, Stower-Hoffmann J, Schneider-Brachert W, Naber KG, Lehn N (2000) Influence of a prophylactic single dose of ciprofloxacin on the level of resistance of Escherichia coli to fluoroquinolones in urology. Int J Antimicrob Agents 15:207–211
13. Carratala J, Fernandez-Sevilla A, Tubau F, Dominguez MA, Gudiol F (1996) Emergence of fluoroquinolone-resistant Escherichia coli in fecal flora of cancer patients receiving norfloxacin prophylaxis. Antimicrob Agents Chemother 40(2):503–505
14. DiBianco JM, Allaway M (2014) Freehand ultrasound-guided transperineal prostate biopsy: technique and early results. J Endourol. doi:10.1089/vid.2014.0046

15. Pepe P, Aragona F (2013) Morbidity after transperineal prostate biopsy in 3000 patients undergoing 12 vs 18 vs more than 24 needle cores. Urology 81:1142–1146
16. Haas GP, Delongchamps N, Brawley OW et al (2008) The worldwide epidemiology of prostate cancer: perspectives from autopsy studies. Can J Urol 15(1):3866–3871
17. Hoogendam A, Buntinx F, devet HC (1999) The diagnostic value of digital rectal examination in primary care screening for prostate cancer: a meta-analysis. Fam Pract 16:621
18. Coley CM, Barry MJ, Fleming C, Mulley AG (1997) Early detection of prostate cancer. Part I: prior probability and effectiveness of tests. The American College of Physicians. Ann Intern Med 126:394
19. Mouraviev V, Lee B, Patel V, Albala D, Johansen TEB, Partin A, Ross A, Perera RJ (2015) Clinical prospects of long noncoding RNAs as novel biomarkers and therapeutic targets in prostate cancer. Prostate Cancer Prostatic Dis. doi:10.1038/pcan.2015.48. [Epub ahead of print]
20. Steensels D et al (2012) Fluoroquinolone-resistant E. coli in intestinal flora of patients undergoing transrectal ultrasound-guided prostate biopsy – should we reassess our practices for antibiotic prophylaxis? Clin Microbiol Infect 18:575–581
21. Bjerklund Johansen TE, Botto H, Cek M et al (2011) Critical review of current definitions of urinary tract infections and proposal of an EAU/ESIU classification system. IJAA 38(Suppl):64–70
22. Bedalov G, Vuckovic I, Fridrich S et al (1994) Prostatitis in benign prostatic hyperplasia: a histological, bacteriological and clinical study. Acta Med Croatica 48:105–109
23. Howard JM, Barker WF, Culbertson WR et al (1964) Postoperative wound infections: the influence of ultraviolet irradiation of the operating room and of various other factors. Ann Surg 160(Suppl):1–192
24. Culver DH, Horan TC, Gaynes RP et al (1991) Surgical wound infection rates by wound class, operative procedure, and patient risk index. Am J Med 91(Suppl 3B):152S–1157S
25. Grabe M, Botto H, Cek M, Tenke P, Wagenlehner FME, Naber KG, Bjerklund Johansen TE (2012) Preoperative assessment of the patient and risk factors for infectious complications and tentative classification of surgical field contamination of urological procedures. World J Urol 30:39–50
26. Jeon SS, Woo SH, Hyun JH, Choi HY, Chai SE (2003) Bisacodyl rectal preparation can decrease infectious complications of transrectal ultrasound-guided prostate biopsy. Urology 62:461–466
27. Abughosh Z, Margolick J, Goldenberg SL (2013) A prospective randomized trial of povidone-iodine prophylactic cleansing of the rectum before transrectal ultrasound guided prostate biopsy. J Urol 189(4):1326–1331. doi:10.1016/j.juro.2012.09.121, Epub 2012 Oct 2
28. Cek M, Tandogdu Z, Naber K, Tenke P, Kristiansen B, Bjerklund Johansen TE (2013) Antimicrobial prophylaxis in urology departments 2005–2010. Eur Urol 63:386–394
29. Wagenlehner FM, Weidner W, Sorgel F, Naber KG (2005) The role of antibiotics in chronic bacterial prostatitis. Int J Antimicrob Agents 26:1–7
30. Naber KG, Sorgel F (2003) Antibiotic therapy – rationale and evidence for optimal drug concentrations in prostatic and seminal fluid and in prostatic tissue. Andrologia 35:331–335
31. Goto T et al (1998) Diffusion of piperacillin, cefotiam, minocycline, amikacin and ofloxacin into the prostate. Int J Urol 5:243–246
32. Naber KG et al (1991) Concentrations of cefpodoxime in plasma, ejaculate and in prostatic fluid and adenoma tissue. Infection 19:30–35
33. Nishikawa G et al (2013) Prostatic penetration of meropenem in humans, and dosage considerations for prostatitis based on a site-specific pharmacokinetic/pharmacodynamic evaluation. Int J Antimicrob Agents 41:267–271
34. Nakamura K et al (2012) Determination of doripenem penetration into human prostate tissue and assessment of dosing regimens for prostatitis based on site-specific pharmacokinetic-pharmacodynamic evaluation. J Chemother 24:32–37
35. Wright WL, Larking P, Lovell-Smith CJ (1982) Concentrations of trimethoprim and sulphamethoxazole in the human prostate gland after intramuscular injection. Br J Urol 54:550–551

36. Jernberg C, Löfmark S, Edlund C, Jansson JK (2010) Long-term impacts of antibiotic expo-
    sure on the human intestinal microbiota. Microbiology 156(Pt 11):3216–3223. doi:10.1099/
    mic.0.040618-0, Epub 2010 Aug 12
37. Wagenlehner FME, Pilatz A, Waliszewski P, Weidner W, Bjerklund-Johansen TE (2014)
    Reducing infection rates during prostate biopsy. Nat Rev Urol 11:80–86. doi:10.1038/
    nrurol.2013.322
38. Kahlmeter G (2003) Prevalence and antimicrobial susceptibility of pathogens in uncompli-
    cated cystitis in Europe. The ECO.SENS study. IJAA 22(Suppl 2):49–52
39. Schaeffer AJ, Weidner W, Barbalias GA et al (2003) Summary, consensus statement: diagnosis
    and management of chronic prostatitis/chronic pelvic pain syndrome. Eur Urol 43(2):1–4

The Contribution of Prostate Infection and Inflammation to BPH and Cancer

10

Francesca Pisano

10.1 Introduction

Although the lower urinary tract symptoms (LUTS) associated with benign prostatic hyperplasia (BPH) are generally due to prostatic enlargement and bladder outlet obstruction (BOO), it is also known that infiltration of inflammatory cells into the prostate plays a role in LUTS development and disease progression [1]. In fact, the presence of inflammatory infiltrates in the prostate biopsy predicted unfavorable outcomes in placebo-treated BPH patients in the Medical Therapy of Prostatic Symptoms (MTOPS) study [2]. Moreover, the Reduction by Dutasteride of Prostate Cancer Events (REDUCE) trial showed that the prevalence of chronic prostatic inflammation in patients with LUTS due to BPH was around 78 % [3]. On the other hand, several epidemiological studies have shown significant association between intraprostatic infiltration of inflammatory cells and prostatic carcinoma. These observations are based on the fact that chronic inflammation and chronic infection influence the emergence of various human neoplasms, such as gastric cancer or bladder cancer related to *Schistosoma haematobium* infection. The mechanism probably is that the inflammatory process causes repeated cell and genome damage which leads to increased cell proliferation (Fig. 10.1).

10.1.1 The Prostate Model

Chronic prostatic inflammation seems to play a crucial role in the pathogenesis and progression of BPH. The remodeling of prostate tissue caused by an inflammatory injury may promote the structural changes that are commonly associated with

F. Pisano
Department of Urology, A.O. Città della Salute e della Scienza, University of Turin, Turin, Italy

Department of Uro-Oncology, Fundaciò Puigvert, Barcelona, Spain
e-mail: francescapisano85@gmail.com

© Springer International Publishing Switzerland 2016
T. Cai, T.E. Bjerklund Johansen (eds.), *Prostatitis and Its Management: Concepts and Recommendations for Clinical Practice*, DOI 10.1007/978-3-319-25175-2_10

Fig. 10.1 Histopathological
evaluation of chronic tissue
inflammatory infiltrate (Courtesy
by Prof Guido Martignoni
(University of Verona, Italy))

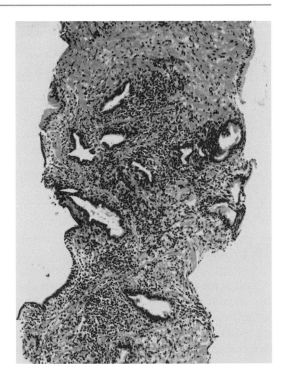

benign disease [4]. The stimulus for prostate inflammatory response in old men is
considered to be multifactorial; potential causes include hormonal changes, infections (bacterial and viral), autoimmune response, urinary reflux inside the prostate,
and systemic inflammation related to metabolic syndrome. Hormonal changes may
promote an increased presence of inflammatory infiltrates in the prostate that could
be responsible for tissue damage both in epithelial and stromal cells. This event can
initiate a chronic process of wound healing which might trigger prostate tissue
remodeling and prostatic enlargement. The effect of inflammation on prostate tissue
is due to the fact that the prostate is an immunocompetent organ populated by a
limited number of inflammatory cells consisting of scattered stromal and intraepithelial T and B lymphocytes, macrophages, and mast cells.

10.1.2 The Prostate: An Immunocompetent Organ

In the adult prostate, a different inflammatory infiltrate pattern has been described
according to the inflammation characteristics. The most common infiltrates are
CD4+ T lymphocytes, CD19 or CD20 B lymphocytes, and macrophages. Regardless
of the trigger, T lymphocytes, macrophages, and B lymphocytes that are [1] present
in the adult prostate can generate damage of both epithelial and stromal cells, stimu-
late cytokine release, and increase the concentration of some growth factors that are
able to promote an abnormal remodeling process characterized by fibromuscular
growth (Fig. 10.2).

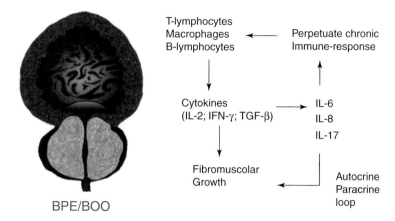

T-lymphocytes
Macrophages   ←——— Perpetuate chronic
B-lymphocytes   Immune-response

Cytokines   ——→   IL-6
(IL-2; IFN-γ; TGF-β)   IL-8
                          IL-17

Fibromuscolar
Growth   ←——   Autocrine
                         Paracrine
BPE/BOO   loop

Fig. 10.2 Role of persistent prostatic inflammation and BPH (Picture taken from De Nunzio et al.)

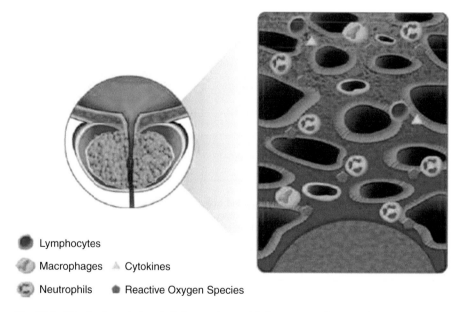

● Lymphocytes

◐ Macrophages   ▲ Cytokines

◉ Neutrophils   ● Reactive Oxygen Species

Fig. 10.3 Distribution of chronic inflammation and inflammatory elements (i.e., lymphocytes, macrophages, neutrophils, cytokines, and ROS) in BHP tissues (Picture taken from Gandaglia et al. [4])

Interleukins and growth factors induce a self-stimulated mechanism characterized by a continuous activation of inflammatory cells, resulting in prostate enlargement. Another leading actor in this pathway is the local hypoxia induced by prostate enlargement itself. As a consequence, reactive oxygen species (ROS) are released and promote neovascularization and further release of growth factors. This mechanism promotes the establishment of a "vicious cycle" that leads to a progressive increase of prostate volume (Figs. 10.3, 10.4, and 10.5).

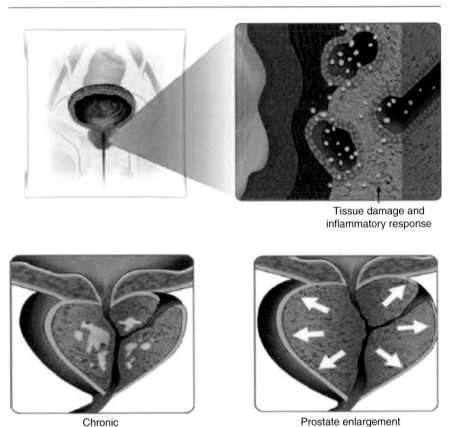

Tissue damage and
inflammatory response

Chronic
process of
wound healing

Prostate enlargement

Fig. 10.4 Representation of the role of chronic prostatic inflammation on BPH pathogenesis. Several stimuli lead to tissue damage, inflammatory response, and the chronic process of wound healing, resulting in prostate enlargement (Picture taken from Gandaglia et al. [4])

10.2 Prostate Inflammation and Prostate Cancer

Prostate cancer (PCa) is the most common cancer in males in Europe. The frequency of incidentally and autopsy-detected cancers is roughly the same in different parts of the world [5]. This finding is in contrast to the incidence of clinical PCa, which differs widely between different geographical areas, being high in the USA and northern Europe. There are some well-established risk factors for PCa: age, ethnic origin, diet, and genetic predisposition. Moreover, the association between prostate inflammation and PCa has already been addressed by various epidemiological studies. Inflammatory cells and ROS produced by immune response mechanisms cause a damage of tissue and genome, as described above. A typical inflammatory infiltrate is usually found in prostate biopsy or in radical prostatectomy specimens. These areas often include prostate cells with a high proliferative index, which is a

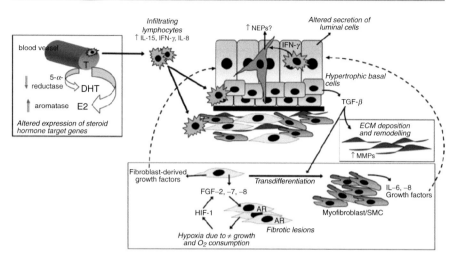

Fig. 10.5 Tissue remodeling in benign prostatic hyperplasia. Global reduction in chromatin methylation may lead to altered gene expression, in particular overexpression of genes regulating cell proliferation and downregulation of genes encoding apoptosis mediators. Age-related changes in systemic sex steroid hormones, together with altered activity of hormone-metabolizing enzymes, lead to an increased intraprostatic estrogen to androgen ratio, which may subsequently alter the expression of steroid hormone-responsive genes. In addition, increased expression of androgen receptor (AR) is observed. Remodeling of the stromal compartment occurs with proliferation of fibroblasts, which secrete growth factors that act on the overlying epithelial compartment, inducing cell proliferation. Increased oxygen consumption of growing tissue may result in local hypoxia with subsequent upregulation of hypoxia-inducible factor-1 (HIF-1) and hypoxia-responsive genes, including FGF-2 and FGF-7. Hypertrophic basal cells actively secrete TGF- β, which induces transdifferentiation of stromal fibroblasts into SMCs and myofibroblasts, which further produce mitogenic growth factors. Increased TGF-β also induces remodeling of the ECM, in particular increased expression of matrix metalloproteinases (MMPs). Altered secretions of luminal cells lead to calcification, clogged ducts, and inflammation. Infiltrating lymphocytes produce inflammatory cytokines, which further promote cell proliferation and differentiation. IFN-γ secreted by invading lymphocytes may induce NE cell differentiation from basal cells and may lead to increased secretion of growth-inducing neuropeptides (NEPs) (Picture taken from Sampson et al. [6])

characteristic aspect of high-grade prostatic intraepithelial neoplasia. As a consequence of this peculiar morphological aspect, these lesions are usually classified as "proliferative inflammatory atrophy" (PIA). PIA is characterized by a very low apoptotic rate, a decreased expression of p27, and hyperproliferation. Morphologically PIA lesions seem to be an intermediate step toward PIN, which is considered as a direct neoplastic precursor. Shah et al. evaluated the distribution of PIA areas in specimens of radical prostatectomy and found that proliferative inflammatory atrophy was significantly more common in the peripheral zone, next to areas of prostatic carcinoma [7]. Moreover these areas seem to present a high nucleic proliferation that is a characteristic aspect of neoplastic degeneration. Concerning the molecular biological aspects, PIA areas usually present an increased expression of glutathione S-transferase P1 (GSTP1) [8]. GSTP1 is involved in the detoxifying process of carcinogens and it is typically overexpressed in inflammatory tissue. A loss of GSTP1 function due to hypermethylation is a common characteristic of prostate cancer cells. Probably a persistent inflammatory state leads to a lack of expression in prostate carcinoma cells. As a consequence, the susceptibility to other genome alterations due to oxidant carcinogens increases and provides a selective growth advantage.

10.3   Genetic Aspects

Genetic predisposition is considered as one of the most important risk factors for developing PCa. If one first-line relative has PCa, the risk is at least doubled. If two or more first-line relatives are affected, the risk increases by 5–11-fold. On the other hand, a small subpopulation of men with prostate cancer (about 9 %) has true hereditary prostate cancer. This is defined as three or more affected relatives or at least two relatives who have developed early-onset disease. Patients with hereditary prostate cancer usually have an onset 6–7 years earlier than spontaneous cases but do not differ in other ways. In order to assess whether or not Mendelian inheritance is involved in the pathogenesis of PCa, some genetic studies have been performed. These analyses of familial prostate carcinoma revealed candidate genes whose products are frequently involved in infectious and inflammatory processes [8].

10.3.1 Chromosome 8p22-23

It contains the macrophage scavenger receptor 1 (MSR 1) gene. Deletions on this chromosome are often detected in hereditary and nonhereditary prostate cancer cells. Mutations at this level are associated with an increased susceptibility to prostate cancer, regardless of the ethnic origin [9]. The analysis of five different variants of this gene in patients with nonhereditary PCa has shown significantly different allele and haplotype frequencies between patients with and without PCa.

10.3.2 Lipopolysaccharide Toll-Like Receptor 4 (TLR4)

It's a crucial element in the pathway of innate immune response to Gram-negative infections. Mutations (single-nucleotide polymorphisms) in the sequence of the gene responsible of its production are associated with a 26 % greater risk of PCa and 39 % greater risk of an early diagnosis (age <65) [10].

10.4   Infections and Prostate Cancer: Which Association?

The role of infections in prostate cancer pathogenesis has been addressed in several studies. The presence of bacterial or viral DNA in prostate cancer cells suggests their potential mutagenic and genotoxic activity [11]. Bacterial RNA gene sequences were found by using PCR in radical prostatectomy specimens and in prostate tissue from patients with BPH [12]. In both groups a strong association between inflammation and positive PCR findings has come to light. Concordance between prostate tissue inflammation and positive PCR results in RP specimens suggests that bacteria might often have a role in histologically inflammatory prostatitis caused by bacteria detectable through their rRNA [13]. The presence of bacterial DNA is a common finding also in patients with chronic pelvic pain syndrome [11]. Bacterial detection rate in this category of patients appears higher than in patients with prostate cancer, confirming the mutagenic role of infections in prostate disease. DNA of viral pathogens was found in prostatic specimens. Its presence seems to be significantly higher in stromal cells, predominantly fibroblasts and hematopoietic elements closer to carcinoma areas, rather than in epithelial cells. This finding should be an expression of the potential role of stromal cells in prostate cancer pathogenesis, by producing proliferative signals or promoting oxidative stress.

10.5 Take-Home Messages and Conclusions

Cell and genome damage and immune system activation induced by infections or other pro-inflammatory stimuli with subsequent inflammation status may play a crucial role in prostate cancer pathogenesis. These considerations may be also used in clinical risk stratification of individuals. Several authors stated that patients with a history of acute prostatitis episodes or with a diagnosis of prostate chronic inflammation should be considered at higher risk of prostate cancer developing. However, these data should be taken with caution until the relationship between prostate tissue inflammation and prostate cancer is better defined. Thus, the identification of patients with chronic inflammation may play a role in the development of treatment targets to prevent BPH progression. In this context, clinical, imaging, and laboratory parameters might be used alone or in combination to identify patients that harbor chronic intraprostatic inflammation.

References

1. Ficarra V, Rossanese M, Zazzara M, GIannarini G, Abbinante M, Bartoletti R, Mirone V, Scaglione F (2014) The role of prostatic inflammation in low urinary tract symptoms (LUTS) due to benign prostatic hyperplasia (BPH) and its potential impact on medical therapy. Curr Urol Rep 15(12):463
2. Roehrborn CG (2008) BPH progression: concept and key learning from MTOPS, ALTESS, COMBAT, and ALF-ONE. BJU Int 101(Suppl 3):17–21
3. Nickel JC, Roherborn CG, O'Leary MP, Bostwick DG, Somerville MC, Rittmaster RS (2008) The relationship between prostate inflammation and lower urinary tract symptoms: examination of baseline data from the REDUCE trial. Eur Urol 54(6):1379–1384
4. Gandaglia G, Briganti A, Gontero P, Mondaini N, Novara G, Salonia A, Sciarra A, Montorsi F (2013) The role of chronic prostatic inflammation in the pathogenesis and progression of benign prostatic hyperplasia (BPH). BJU Int 112(4):432–441
5. Heidenreich A, Bastian PJ, Bellmunt J, Bolla M, Joniau S, van der Kwast T, Mason M, Matveev V, Wiegel T, Zattoni F, Mottet N (2013). EAU guidelines on prostate cancer,

part 1: screening, diagnosis and local treatment with curative intent-update. Eur Urol 65(1):124–37

6. Sampson N, Untergasser G, Plas E, Berger P (2007) The ageing male reproductive tract. J Pathol 211(2):206–218

7. Shah R, Mucci NR, Amin A, Macoska JA, Rubin MA (2001) Postatrophic hyperplasia of the prostate gland: neoplastic precursor or innocent bystander? Am J Pathol 158(5):1767–1773

8. Wagenlehner FME, Elkahwaji JE, Algaba F, Bjerklund-Johansen T, Naber KG, Hartung R, Weidner W (2007) The role of inflammation and infection in the pathogenesis of prostate carcinoma. BJU Int 100(4):733–737

9. Xu J, Zheng SL, Komiya A et al (2003) Common sequence variants of the macrophage scavenger receptor 1 gene are associated with prostate cancer risk. Am J Hum Genet 72(1):208–212

10. Zheng SL, Augustsson-Balter K, Chang B et al (2004) Sequence variants of toll-like receptor 4 are associated with prostate cancer risk: results from the Cancer Prostate in Sweden Study. Cancer Res 64:2918–2922

11. Krieger JN, Riley DE, Vesella RL, Miner DC, Ross SO, Lange PH (2000) Bacterial DNA sequences in prostate tissue from patients with prostate cancer and chronic prostatitis. J Urol 164(4):1221–1228

12. Nickel JC, Downey J, Hunter D, Clark J (2001) Prevalence of prostatitis-like symptoms in a population based study using the National Institutes of Health chronic prostatitis symptom index. J Urol 165(3):842–845

13. Hochreiter WW, Duncan JL, Schaeffer AJ (2000) Evaluation of the bacterial flora of the prostate using a 16S rRNA gene based polymerase chain reaction. J Urol 163(1):127–130

The Role of STD Pathogens in Bacterial Prostatitis

11

Tommaso Cai and Daniele Tiscione

11.1 *Chlamydia trachomatis* Infections

11.1.1 Microbiological Considerations

Chlamydia trachomatis is an obligate intracellular Gram-negative bacterium that needs living cells to multiply due to its inability to synthesize essential nutrients and depends on host biosynthesis pathways (Fig. 11.1) [1].

Chlamydia trachomatis has been divided into several different serotypes on the basis of their major outer membrane protein (MOMP) characteristics. Serotypes A, B, and C are the causes of trachoma; serotypes D through K cause urogenital infections, and serotype L is responsible for lymphogranuloma venereum [1–3].

Chlamydia trachomatis shows two phases of reproduction:

1. An intracellular phase of noninfectious metabolically active and replicative reticular bodies (RBs)
2. An extracellular phase of infectious metabolically inactive and non-replicative elementary bodies (EBs) [4, 5]

The biphasic developmental cycle of *Chlamydia trachomatis* consists of the conversion of EBs to RBs, followed by RB cell division and transformation back to infective EBs. EBs then infect epithelial cells by means of several potential receptors including PRRs, followed by endocytosis, which leads to the formation of membrane-bound, glycogen-enriched intracellular inclusions [1]. Once inside the epithelial cells, *Chlamydia trachomatis* undergoes the conversion to RBs in order to

T. Cai • D. Tiscione (✉)
Department of Urology, Santa Chiara Regional Hospital, Trento, Italy
e-mail: ktommy@libero.it; daniele.tiscione@apss.tn.it

© Springer International Publishing Switzerland 2016
T. Cai, T.E. Bjerklund Johansen (eds.), *Prostatitis and Its Management: Concepts and Recommendations for Clinical Practice*, DOI 10.1007/978-3-319-25175-2_11

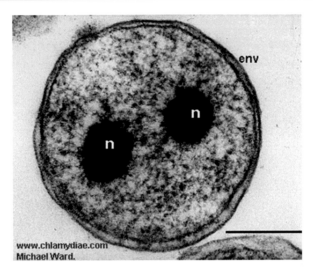

Fig. 11.1 An intermediate body of *Chlamydia trachomatis* undergoing differentiation. In this figure there are two points of condensation of DNA into electron-dense nucleoids (*n*). Note the inner cytoplasmic membrane and the outer envelope (*env*) (Image taken from http://chlamydiae.com/twiki/images/ArchiveDocsBiologyBiolRB_4.gif)

replicate and finally converts again to infective EBs, which infect neighboring epithelial cells. These EBs are released after host cell lysis and can survive in the extracellular environment as infectious agents [1, 4, 6]. After lysis of the infected host cells, mucosal epithelial cells undergo necrosis [1] (Fig. 11.2).

During the infection cycle, all chlamydial components, such as the endotoxin lipopolysaccharide (LPS) and bacterial proteins, activate the host immune response [1]. Neutrophils, monocytes, dendritic cells, lymphocytes, and plasma B cells migrate into this necrotic and ulcerous epithelium [1, 7, 8]. Local inflammation can lead to fibrosis followed by the shriveling of connective tissue structures and scarring [1] (Fig. 11.3).

11.1.2 Epidemiological Considerations

Chlamydia trachomatis is the most common sexually transmitted bacterium worldwide, with over three million new infections per year [9, 10]. The World Health Organization estimates that 92 million new cases of Ct occur worldwide every year [11]. In particular, *Chlamydia trachomatis* is the most frequently reported sexually transmitted infection in Europe, and the number of cases is steadily increasing, with more than 25,5000 cases in people below 25 years of age [12] (Fig. 11.4).

The rate of transmission between sexual partners may be as high as 75 % [13]. However, approximately 75 % of *Chlamydia trachomatis* infections in women and up to 50 % of those in men are asymptomatic [14, 15]. This aspect is extremely

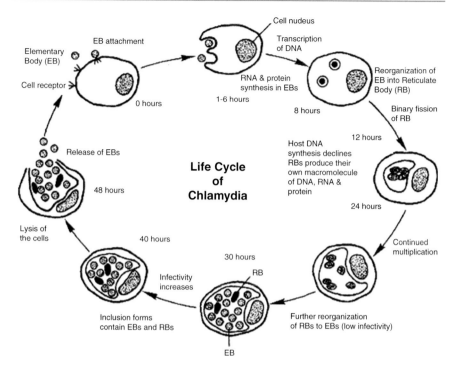

Fig. 11.2 The *Chlamydia trachomatis* life cycle (Image taken from http://www.tutorsglobe.com/homework-help/microbiology/chlamydia-72780.aspx)

Fig. 11.3 A colorized scanning electron micrograph shows a cultured human cell infected by *Chlamydia trachomatis*, appearing as small round particles inside the cell wall (Image taken from http://abcnews.go.com/Health/chlamydia-outbreak-hits-texas-high-school-sex-ed/story?id=30798143)

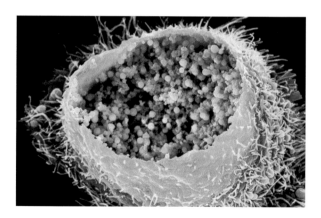

important due to the fact that although up to 13.3 % of young men may have a genital chlamydial infection, only half of these will present with any symptoms, and even fewer are likely to pursue treatment [16]. Moreover, the absence of symptoms increases the risk of infecting sexual partners and may also cause long-term complications in men, such as poor semen quality and infertility [17–19].

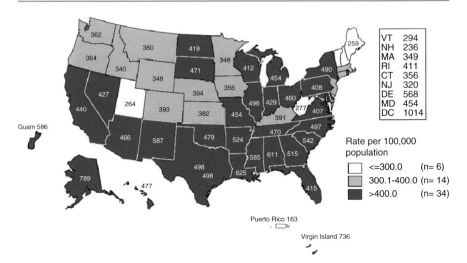

VT 294
NH 236
MA 349
RI 411
CT 356
NJ 320
DE 568
MD 454
DC 1014

Guam 586

Rate per 100,000
population

☐ <=300.0   (n= 6)
▨ 300.1-400.0 (n= 14)
■ >400.0   (n= 34)

Puerto Rico 163

Virgin Island 736

Fig. 11.4 *Chlamydia trachomatis*—Rates of Reported Cases by State, United States and Outlying Areas, 2013 – the total rate of reported cases of *Chlamydia trachomatis* for the United States and outlying areas (Guam, Puerto Rico, and Virgin Islands) was 443.5 per 100,000 population (Image taken from the Sexually Transmitted Disease Surveillance 2013 – Division of STD Prevention December 2014 – U.S. DEPARTMENT OF HEALTH AND HUMAN SERVICES – Centers for Disease Control and Prevention – National Center for HIV/AIDS, Viral Hepatitis, STD, and TB Prevention – Division of STD Prevention – Atlanta, Georgia 30333 (http://www.cdc.gov/std/stats13/surv2013-print.pdf))

11.1.3 Clinical Presentation in Men

In men, *Chlamydia trachomatis* is responsible for urethritis, epididymitis, orchitis, and prostatitis [20–22]. In addition, *Chlamydia trachomatis* infection has been reported to be a major cause of reactive arthritis [23]. Furthermore, it has been shown that 21 % of patients with unexplained arthritis have a history of urogenital chlamydial infection [24, 25]. On the other hand, the consequences of *Chlamydia trachomatis* infection for male fertility are still under debate, with some reports arguing no effect on male fertility and others reporting decreased semen quality and impaired sperm fertilizing capacity and DNA integrity [26–28]. However, the most common clinical presentation is an asymptomatic infection [1]. In fact, although *Chlamydia trachomatis* induces local inflammation and triggers the host immune response, infection remains subclinical in most infected individuals [1, 29]. Several times patients present with mucopurulent discharge, dysuria, and pruritus 1–3 weeks after intercourse (Fig. 11.5).

The factors that determine whether infections develop as symptomatic or asymptomatic are unknown. However, a high prevalence of serotype E and its lack of associated clinical symptoms may suggest that this serotype might be more successful in maintaining a subclinical infection than other, less prevalent serotypes. Indeed, a successful serotype would be one that remains undetected for a longer period of time, enhancing dissemination. Variability of the main Ct antigen MOMP is

Fig. 11.5 Urethral
discharge

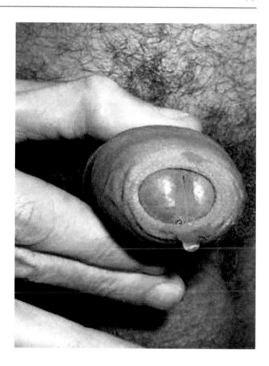

presumably the result of host selection and bacterial adaptation [1]. Thus, the
MOMP sequence that elicits a milder immune response in the infected host could be
an adaptive mode of evolution to escape immune pressure and might therefore confer a transmission advantage over other MOMP serotypes [1].

As a consequence, little attention has been paid to *Chlamydia trachomatis* infection of the male genital tract, as it is underestimated and mainly considered to be a
reservoir for transmission and reinfection [1, 30]. Although in men *Chlamydia trachomatis* mainly affects the urethra and epididymis, it has also been reported to
infect other tissues such as the prostate and seminal vesicles [1, 31, 32]. Here, we
will focus on prostatic infection.

11.1.4 Chronic Prostatitis

In males, after the first infection of the single-cell columnar layer of the urethral
epithelium, *Chlamydia trachomatis* infects nearby epithelial cells leading to an
ascending infection and can cause retrograde epididymitis and epididymo-orchitis
[1, 33, 34]. Moreover, the ascending infection from the urethra can reach the prostate epithelium and cause prostate and seminal vesicle infections [1, 32, 33]
(Fig. 11.6).

Even if chronic prostatitis/chronic pelvic pain syndrome (CPPS) is the most
common prostatitis syndrome, constituting 90–95 % of prostatitis cases, the CPPS
etiology and pathogenesis are uncertain [35]. The etiology of CPPS remains

Fig. 11.6 Ascending infection
from urethra to prostate and
seminal vesicles

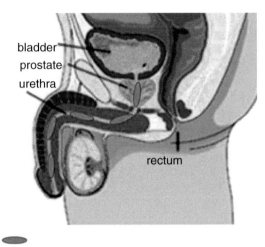

Chlamydia trachomatis

unknown and few hypotheses are currently under consideration. One such hypothesis postulates a microbial etiology due to a cryptic undetected microbial pathogen, suggesting that these patients should be classified as having bacterial prostatitis [1, 35]. In this regard, several studies have focused on *Chlamydia trachomatis* as an etiological agent of CPPS [3, 36–38].

For diagnostic purposes, microbiological analysis, as well as evaluation of the presence of leukocytes, is performed in expressed prostatic secretion, semen, and/or urine pre- and post-prostatic massage samples [1]. After negative conventional microbiological cultures, physicians perform microbiological, cell culture, or molecular tests for diagnosis of specific pathogens [1]. Assays to detect antibodies specific for microorganisms in seminal plasma and serum may be valid for seroepidemiological studies, but not for diagnostic purposes [39]. The cross-reactivity of antibodies between *Chlamydia trachomatis* and some *Chlamydophila* species and the persistence of antibody titers over time impair the possibility of performing an accurate diagnosis and make it difficult to distinguish between past and current infections [40].

The prevalence of *Chlamydia trachomatis* infection in CP/CPPS patients has been reported to range from 8.3 to 27 % [1]. Some authors have raised concerns about the reliability of the samples used in these studies [37]. They postulated that bacterial isolation from prostate diagnostic material presents a potential risk of contamination while going through the urethra, thus limiting the interpretation of the test [37]. However, a number of studies indicate that semen/expressed prostatic secretion specimens are often positive for *Chlamydia trachomatis* in patients with negative urethral swabs [41, 42]. Also, pure prostatic biopsies from CP/CPPS have demonstrated the presence of *Chlamydia trachomatis* in the absence of urethral infection [32]. These findings undoubtedly support the role of *Chlamydia trachomatis* as a causative or triggering agent of CP/CPPS.

11.1.5 *Chlamydia trachomatis* Infection of the Prostate Epithelium: What Are the Consequences?

Chlamydia trachomatis infection of the prostate gland may cause inflammation within the prostatic tissue, thus impairing the normal functionality of the gland, and as is well known, prostate secretions account for up to 60 % of the volume of seminal plasma [43].

11.1.5.1 Reduction of Volume of Seminal Plasma

The main function of the prostate gland is the production of large amounts of soluble proteins and components that are secreted into the ejaculate [1]. These proteins optimize the conditions for successful fertilization, providing an adequate medium for the survival of sperm and enhancing sperm motility in the female reproductive tract [1, 44]. It could be speculated that an inflammation of the prostate gland due to *Chlamydia trachomatis* infection will alter the gland function and thereby impair male fertility.

11.1.5.2 Alteration of Semen Quality

As stated above, the literature concerning this issue is controversial, with some reports arguing in favor of a positive relationship between chronic prostatitis caused by *Chlamydia trachomatis* and altered semen quality [28, 45], whereas other reports support the idea that no alterations are produced in semen quality and male fertility [31]. An important feature is the chronic nature of this infection and also the recruitment of immune cells that in turn produce a local but mild inflammation that remains subclinical in most infected individuals [1]. Whether or not urethritis, vesiculitis, prostatitis, epididymitis, and orchitis caused by *Chlamydia trachomatis* lead to significant detrimental effects on male fertility for certain is still controversial [46].

11.1.6 The Management of the Patient

The clinical management of *Chlamydia trachomatis* infection should include:

1. Treatment of patients (to reduce complications and prevent transmission to sex partners)
2. Treatment of sex partners (to prevent reinfection of the index patient and infection of other partners)
3. Risk-reduction counseling
4. Repeat chlamydial testing in women a few months after treatment (to identify recurrent/persistent infections) [47, 48]

The indications for treatment are:

1. Confirmed genital *Chlamydia trachomatis* infection
2. Infection with *Chlamydia trachomatis* in the partner

3. In a patient with a confirmed *Neisseria gonorrhoeae* infection if laboratory tests for *Chlamydia trachomatis* are not available
4. In a patient with clinical signs of a chlamydial infection if laboratory tests for *Chlamydia trachomatis* are not available [49]

On the basis of clinical presentation or on the results of the laboratory examinations, we consider three clinical settings:

1. Patient with urethral infection
2. Patient with prostate infection
3. Infertile patient with prostatitis due to *Chlamydia trachomatis* infection

11.1.7 Patient with Urethral Infection

First-line regimens include azithromycin 1 g orally as a single dose or doxycycline 100 mg orally twice a day for 7 days. Several alternative regimens have been proposed: erythromycin base 500 mg orally four times a day for 7 days, ofloxacin 200 mg orally twice a day for 7 days, roxithromycin 150 mg orally twice a day for 7 days, clarithromycin 250 mg orally twice a day for 7 days, levofloxacin 500 mg once daily for 7 days, or ofloxacin 300 mg twice a day for 7 days [49]. In cases of rectal non-lymphogranuloma venereum chlamydial infections, the first choice should be a course of doxycycline, 100 mg twice daily for 7 days [49, 50].

11.1.8 Patient with Prostate Infection

There are few published trials about the therapy of prostatitis due to *Chlamydia trachomatis* infection. Recently, Cai et al. evaluated the efficacy of a 14-day course of prulifloxacin 600 mg with standard antibiotic therapy (doxycycline 100 mg twice daily for 21 days) for the treatment of chronic prostatitis due to *Chlamydia trachomatis* infection [51]. By using a non-inferiority RCT, they concluded that prulifloxacin is equivalent to standard therapy regarding clinical success, as demonstrated by a decrease in the number of patients affected by CP due to *Chlamydia trachomatis* infection [51]. Recently, Miyashita et al. demonstrated the efficacy of a new-generation fluoroquinolone, sitafloxacin, against *Chlamydia trachomatis* infection [52]. Its antimicrobial activity is unique compared to conventional fluoroquinolones, although few clinical studies have been reported [53, 54].

11.1.9 The Infertile Patient with Prostatitis Due to *Chlamydia trachomatis* Infection

It is well known that chronic prostatitis due to *Chlamydia trachomatis* infection not only decreases the quality of life [55] but also has a significant impact on a couple's reproductive health [28]. Indeed, *Chlamydia trachomatis* has a significant role in male infertility, and eradication of the infection is critical for the recovery of the man's fertility [56]. However, eradication of the infection after antibiotic therapy does not always result in recovery of semen quality, and other treatment compounds may be needed. Recently, Cai et al., using a prospective, randomized, and controlled study, demonstrated that L-arginine, L-carnitine, acetyl-L-carnitine, and ginseng extracts, together with prulifloxacin, improved semen parameters in patients with *Chlamydia trachomatis* genital infection and oligoasthenoteratozoospermia compared to treatment with prulifloxacin therapy alone [57]. The improved quality of spermatozoa from an infertile status to a normal fertility index was demonstrated by two sets of findings. The anti-inflammatory and antioxidative effects of ginseng improved the shape and concentration of spermatozoa, and L-arginine, L-carnitine, and acetyl-L-carnitine enhanced sperm motility and function by stimulating the activity of endothelial nitric oxide synthase [57–59]. Two important aspects in the treatment of male infertility in patients affected by chronic prostatitis and oligoasthenoteratozoospermia due to *Chlamydia trachomatis* infection should be discussed. Firstly, specific treatment of infertility should be started concurrently with the antibiotic treatment. Then, the association of antibiotic therapy with L-arginine, L-carnitine, acetyl-L-carnitine, and ginseng extracts together can produce good results in terms of recovery of semen quality [57].

11.1.10 Treatment Failure

A repeated course or a longer course (10–14 days) with doxycycline or a macrolide has been suggested, but evidence is lacking [49]. The most common reason for therapy failure is reinfection from an untreated partner [49, 60]. An interesting suggestion is the combined use of rifampicin and a macrolide [61]. Finally, the potential of *Chlamydia trachomatis* to develop antimicrobial resistance has not been well studied, although some case reports suggest resistance as a cause of treatment failure [62, 63].

11.1.11 Coinfections with Other Sexually Transmitted Infections

Men and women with a diagnosis of *Chlamydia trachomatis* infection should be offered a complete workup for other sexually transmitted infections, such as gonorrhea, syphilis, mycoplasmata, human papillomavirus, and HIV [19, 49]. If coinfection with *Mycoplasma genitalium* is confirmed, patients should not be treated with a single dose of 1 g azithromycin, but with a short course of azithromycin: 500 mg on day 1 followed by 250 mg on days 2–5 [49, 64].

11.2   Mycoplasmata Infections

11.2.1 Microbiological and Clinical Considerations

Mycoplasma infections affect the cellular metabolism and physiology of the host organism and are associated with diseases in humans and animals [65, 66]. In males the most frequent strains found in the urogenital tract are *Mycoplasma hominis*,

Mycoplasma genitalium, and *Ureaplasma urealyticum*. However, their role in urogenital tract infections remains unknown. In fact, these Mollicutes present a complex relationship with the host immune response, and several times they can be considered as normal commensals of the human urogenital microflora which only become pathogenic under specific, relatively rare conditions [65, 66]. Even if *Ureaplasma urealyticum* may cause non-chlamydial urethritis, the role in prostate infection is totally unknown. *Mycoplasma genitalium* has been isolated from urethral swab samples, but studies attempting to assess its association with disease were hampered by difficulties to grow the organism in culture [67, 68]. However, in recent years, a more reliable detection became possible after the development of specific PCR assays. Subsequent studies that used these assays have provided strong evidence of an association between acute urethritis in heterosexual men and *Mycoplasma genitalium* [69]. However, up to the moment there is no significant data supporting the role of mycoplasma in prostate infection. In case of coinfection with other sexually transmitted diseases, the suggested therapy is a short course of azithromycin: 500 mg on day 1 followed by 250 mg on days 2–5 [49, 64].

References

1. Wyrick PB (2000) Intracellular survival by Chlamydia. Cell. Microbiol 2:275–282 – Chlamydia trachomatis infection of the male genital tract: an updateJuan; updateJuan Pablo Mackern-Obertia, Rubén Darío Motricha, María Laura Bresera,Leonardo Rodolfo Sáncheza, Cecilia Cuffinib, Virginia Elena Riveroa
2. Brunham RC, Rey-Ladino J (2005) Immunology of Chlamydia infection: implications for a Chlamydia trachomatis vaccine. Nat Rev Immunol 5:149–161
3. Wagenlehner FME, Naber KG, Weidner W (2006) Chlamydial infec-tions and prostatitis in men. BJU Int 97:687–690
4. Schachter J, Stephens RS (2008) Biology of Chlamydia trachomatis. In: Holmes KK, Sparling PF, Stamm WE (eds) Sexually transmitted diseases. McGraw-Hill Companies, Inc, New York, pp 555–574
5. Valdivia RH (2008) Chlamydia effector proteins and new insights into chlamydial cellular microbiology. Curr Opin Microbiol 11:53–59
6. Witkin SS (2002) Immunological aspects of genital chlamydia infections. Best Pract Res Clin Obstet Gynaecol 16:865–874
7. Agrawal T, Vats V, Salhan S, Mittal A (2009) The mucosal immune response to Chlamydia trachomatis infection of the reproductive tractin women. J Reprod Immunol 83:173–178
8. Al-Zeer MA, Al-Younes HM, Braun PR, Zerrahn J, Meyer TF (2009) IFN-γ-inducible irga6 mediates host resistance against Chlamydia tra-chomatis via autophagy. PLoS One 4:e4588
9. Cai T, Mazzoli S, Mondaini N, Malossini G, Bartoletti R (2011) Chlamydia trachomatis infection: a challenge for the urologist. Microbiol Res 2, e14. doi:10.4081/mr.2011.e14
10. Groseclose SL, Zaidi AA, DeLisle SJ, Levine WC, St Louis ME (1999) Estimated incidence and prevalence of genital Chlamydia trachomatis infections in the United States, 1996. Sex Transm Dis 26:339–344, PMID: 10417022
11. World Health Organization. Global prevalence and incidence of selected curable sexually transmitted infections: overview and estimates. Available from: URL: http://whqlibdoc.who.int/hq/2001/WHO_HIV_AIDS_2001.02.pdf. Accessed 15 Jul 2010
12. European Centre for Disease Prevention and Control. Most common STI in Europe. Available from: URL: http://www.ecdc.europa.eu/en/healthtopics/spotlight/chlamydia/Pages/KeyMessage1.aspx

13. Markos AR (2005) The concordance of Chlamydia trachomatis genital infection between sexual partners, in the era of nucleic acid testing. Sex Health 2:23–24, PMID: 16334709
14. Gonzales GF, Muñoz G, Sánchez R, Henkel R, Gallegos-Avila G, Díaz-Gutierrez O, Vigil P, Vásquez F, Kortebani G, Mazzolli A, Bustos-Obregón E (2004) Update on the impact of Chlamydia trachomatis infection on male fertility. Andrologia 36:1–23, PMID: 14871260
15. Stamm WE (1999) Chlamydia trachomatis infections: progress and problems. J Infect Dis 179(Suppl 2):S380–S383, PMID:10081511
16. LaMontagne DS, Fenton KA, Randall S, Anderson S, Carter P (2004) Establishing the National Chlamydia Screening Programme in England: results from the first full year of screening. Sex Transm Infect 80:335–341, PMID: 15459399
17. Mazzoli S, Cai T, Addonisio P, Bechi A, Mondaini N, Bartoletti R (2010) Chlamydia trachomatis infection is related to poor semen quality in young prostatitis patients. Eur Urol 57:708–714 [PMID: 19482415, doi:10.1016/j.eururo.2009.05.015]
18. Park IU, Amey A, Creegan L, Barandas A, Bauer HM (2010) Retesting for repeat chlamydial infection: family planning provider knowledge, attitudes, and practices. J Womens Health (Larchmt) 19:1139–1144 [PMID: 20482236, doi:10.1089/jwh.2009.1648]
19. Cai T, Wagenlehner FM, Mondaini N, D'Elia C, Meacci F, Migno S, Malossini G, Mazzoli S, Bartoletti R (2014) Effect of human papillomavirus and Chlamydia trachomatis co-infection on sperm quality in young heterosexual men with chronic prostatitis-related symptoms. BJU Int 113(2):281–287
20. Cunningham KA, Beagley KW (2008) Male genital tract chlamydial infection: implications for pathology and infertility. Biol Reprod 79:180–189
21. Ouzounova-Raykova V, Ouzounova I, Mitov IG (2010) Chlamydia tra-chomatis be an aetiological agent of chronic prostatic infection? Andrologia 42:176–181
22. Kalwij S, French S, Mugezi R, Baraitser P (2012) Using educational outreach and a financial incentive to increase general practices' con-tribution to chlamydia screening in South-East London 2003–2011. BMC Public Health 12:802
23. Carter JD, Hudson AP (2010) The evolving story of Chlamydia-induced reactive arthritis. Curr Opin Rheumatol 22:424–430
24. Wollenhaupt J, Kolbus F, Weissbrodt H, Schneider C, Krech T, Zeidler H (1995) Manifestations of Chlamydia induced arthritis in patients with silent versus symptomatic urogenital chlamydial infection. Clin Exp Rheumatol 13:453–458
25. Senior K (2012) Chlamydia: a much underestimated STI. Lancet Infect Dis 12:517–518
26. Paavonen J, Eggert-Kruse W (1999) Chlamydia trachomatis: impact on human reproduction. Hum Reprod Update 5:433–447
27. Joki-Korpela P, Sahrakorpi N, Halttunen M, Surcel H-M, Paavonen J, Tiitinen A (2009) The role of Chlamydia trachomatis infection in male infertility. Fertil Steril 91:1448–1450
28. Mazzoli S, Cai T, Addonisio P, Bechi A, Mondaini N, Bartoletti R (2010) Chlamydia trachomatis infection is related to poor semen quality in young prostatitis patients. Eur Urol 57:708–714
29. Gottlieb SL, Berman SM, Low N (2010) Screening and treatment to pre-vent sequelae in women with Chlamydia trachomatis genital infection:how much do we know? J Infect Dis 201:156–167
30. Chen MY, Basil D (2003) Screening for genital Chlamydia trachomatis infection: are men the forgotten reservoir? Med J Aust 179:124–125
31. Motrich RD, Cuffini C, Mackern Oberti JP, Maccioni M, Rivero VE (2006) Chlamydia trachomatis occurrence and its impact on sperm qual-ity in chronic prostatitis patients. J Infect 53:175–183
32. Toth M, Patton DL, Campbell LA, Carretta EI, Mouradian J, Toth A, Shevchuk M, Baergen R, Ledger W (2000) Detection of chlamydial antigenic material in ovarian, prostatic, ectopic pregnancy and semen samples of culture-negative subjects. Am J Reprod Immunol 43:218–222
33. Krishnan R, Heal M (1991) Study of the seminal vesicles in acute epi-didymitis. Br J Urol 67:632–637

34. Trojian TH, Lishmak T, Heiman SD (2009) Epididymitis and orchitis:an overview. Am Fam Physician 79:583–587
35. Habermacher GM, Chason JT, Schaeffer AJ (2006) Prostatitis/chronic pelvic pain syndrome. Annu Rev Med 57:195–206
36. Mazzoli S, Cai T, Rupealta V, Gavazzi A, Castricchi Pagliai R, Mondaini N, Bartoletti R (2007) Interleukin 8 and anti-chlamydia trachomatis mucosal IgA as urogenital immunologic markers in patients with C. trachomatis prostatic infection. Eur Urol 51(5):1385–1393
37. Weidner W, Diemer T, Huwe P, Rainer H, Ludwig M (2002) The role of Chlamydia trachomatis in prostatitis. Int J Antimicrob Agents 19:466–470
38. Motrich RD, Maccioni M, Riera CM, Rivero VE (2007) Autoimmuneprostatitis: state of the art. Scand J Immunol 66:217–227
39. Taylor-Robinson D (1997) Evaluation and comparison of tests to diag-nose Chlamydia trachomatis genital infections. Hum Reprod 12:113–120
40. Gijsen AP, Land JA, Goossens VJ, Leffers P, Bruggeman CA, Evers JLH (2001) Chlamydia pneumoniae and screening for tubal factor subfertility. Hum Reprod 16:487–491
41. Corradi G, Konkoly Thege M, Pánovics J, Molnár G, Bodó A, Frang D (1995) Is seminal fluid a suitable specimen for detecting chlamydial infection in men? Acta Microbiol Immunol Hung 42:389–394
42. Skerk V, Krhen I, Schonwald S, Cajic V, Markovinovic L, Roglic S, Zekan S, Andracevic AT, Kruzic V (2004) The role of unusual pathogens in prostatitis syndrome. Int J Antimicrob Agents 24:53–56
43. Lepor H, Lawson RK (1994) Enfermedades de la próstata. Editorial Panamericana, Buenos Aires
44. Elzanaty S, Richthoff J, Malm J, Giwercman A (2002) The impact of epididymal and accessory sex gland function on sperm motility. Hum Reprod 17:2904–2911
45. La Vignera S, Vicari E, Condorelli RA, D'Agata R, Calogero AE (2011) Male accessory gland infection and sperm parameters (review). Int J Androl 34:e330–e347
46. Weidner W, Ludwig M, Thiele D, Floren E, Zimmermann O (1996) Chlamydial antibodies in semen: Search for "silent" chlamydial infec-tions in asymptomatic andrological patients. Infection 24:309–313
47. Geisler WM (2007) Management of uncomplicated Chlamydia trachomatis infections in adolescents and adults: evidence reviewed for the 2006 Centers for Disease Control and Prevention sexually transmitted diseases treatment guidelines. Clin Infect Dis 44(Suppl 3):S77–S83
48. Lee YS, Lee KS (2013) Chlamydia and male lower urinary tract diseases. Korean J Urol 54:73–77
49. Lanjouw E, Ossewaarde JM, Stary A, Boag F, van der Meijden WI (2010) 2010 European guideline for the management of Chlamydia trachomatis infections. Int J STD AIDS 21:729–737
50. de Vries HJ, Smelov V, Middelburg JG, Pleijster J, Speksnijder AG, Morré SA (2009) Delayed microbial cure of lymphogranuloma venereum proctitis with doxycycline treatment. Clin Infect Dis 48:e53–e56
51. Cai T, Mazzoli S, Addonisio P, Boddi V, Geppetti P, Bartoletti R (2010) Clinical and microbiological efficacy of prulifloxacin for the treatment of chronic bacterial prostatitis due to Chlamydia trachomatis infection: results from a prospective, randomized and open-label study. Methods Find Exp Clin Pharmacol 32:39–45
52. Miyashita N, Niki Y, Matsushima T (2001) In vitro and in vivo activities of sitafloxacin against Chlamydia spp. Antimicrob Agents Chemother 45:3270–3272
53. Sato K, Hoshino K, Tanaka M, Hayakawa I, Osada Y (1992) Antimicrobial activity of DU-6859, a new potent fluoroquinolone, against clinical isolates. Antimicrob Agents Chemother 36:1491–1498
54. Takahashi S, Hamasuna R, Yasuda M, Ito S, Ito K, Kawai S, Yamaguchi T, Satoh T, Sunaoshi K, Takeda K, Suzuki N, Maeda S, Nishimura H, Fukuda S, Matsumoto T (2013) Clinical efficacy of sitafloxacin 100 mg twice daily for 7 days for patients with nongonococcal urethritis. J Infect Chemother 19:941–945

55. Walz J, Perrotte P, Hutterer G, Suardi N, Jeldres C, Bénard F, Valiquette L, Karakiewicz PI (2007) Impact of chronic prostatitis like symptoms on the quality of life in a large group of men. BJU Int 100:1307–1311

56. Ochsendorf FR, Ozdemir K, Rabenau H, Fenner T, Oremek R, Milbradt R, Doerr HW (1999) Chlamydia trachomatis and male infertility: chlamydia-IgA antibodies in seminal plasma are C. trachomatis specific and associated with an inflammatory response. J Eur Acad Dermatol Venereol 12:143–152

57. Cai T, Wagenlehner FM, Mazzoli S, Meacci F, Mondaini N, Nesi G, Tiscione D, Malossini G, Bartoletti R (2012) Semen quality in patients with Chlamydia trachomatis genital infection treated concurrently with prulifloxacin and a phytotherapeutic agent. J Androl 33:615–623

58. Saw CL, Wu Q, Kong AN (2010) Anti-cancer and potential chemopreventive actions of ginseng by activating Nrf2 (NFE2L2) anti-oxidative stress/anti-inflammatory pathways. Chin Med 5:37

59. Stanislavov R, Nikolova V, Rohdewald P (2009) Improvement of seminal parameters with Prelox: a randomized, doubleblind, placebo-controlled, cross-over trial. Phytother Res 23:297–302

60. Batteiger BE, Tu W, Ofner S, Van Der Pol B, Stothard DR, Orr DP, Katz BP, Fortenberry JD (2010) Repeated Chlamydia trachomatis genital infections in adolescent women. J Infect Dis 201:42–51

61. Dreses-Werringloer U, Padubrin I, Zeidler H, Köhler L (2001) Effects of azithromycin and rifampin on Chlamydia trachomatis infection in vitro. Antimicrob Agents Chemother 45:3001–3008

62. Somani J, Bhullar VB, Workowski KA, Farshy CE, Black CM (2000) Multiple drug-resistant Chlamydia trachomatis associated with clinical treatment failure. J Infect Dis 181:1421–1427

63. Mourad A, Sweet RL, Sugg N, Schachter J (1980) Relative resistance to erythromycin in Chlamydia trachomatis. Antimicrob Agents Chemother 18:696–698

64. Björnelius E, Anagrius C, Bojs G, Carlberg H, Johannisson G, Johansson E, Moi H, Jensen JS, Lidbrink P (2008) Antibiotic treatment of symptomatic Mycoplasma genitalium infection in Scandinavia: a controlled clinical trial. Sex Transm Infect 84:72–76

65. Razin S, Yogev D, Naot Y (1998) Molecular biology and pathogenicity of mycoplasmas. Microbiol Mol Biol Rev 62:1094–1156

66. Sun G, Xu X, Wang Y, Shen X, Chen Z, Yang J (2008) Mycoplasma pneumoniae infection induces reactive oxygen species and DNA damage in A549 human lung carcinoma cells. Infect Immun 76:4405–4413

67. Palmer HM, Gilroy CB, Furr PM, Taylor-Robinson D (1991) Development of evaluation of the polymerase chain reaction to detect Mycoplasma genitalium. FEMS Microbiol Lett 61:199–203

68. Jensen JS, Uldum SA, Søndergård-Anderson J et al (1991) Polymerase chain reaction for detection of Mycoplasma genitalium in clinical samples. J Clin Microbiol 29:46–50

69. Mena L, Wang X, Mroczkowski TF, Martin DH (2002) Mycoplasma genitalium infections in asymptomatic men and men with urethritis attending a sexually transmitted diseases clinic in New Orleans. Clin Infect Dis 35(10):1167–1173

Andrologic Sequelae in Prostatitis Patients

12

Jamil Syed and Vladimir Mouraviev

12.1 Introduction

Chronic prostatitis/chronic pelvic pain syndrome (CP/CPPS) is the most prevalent of the four categories of prostatitis. CP/CPPS is also the form of prostatitis that has been most associated with andrologic sequelae. Hypogonadism and sexual dysfunction have both been implicated to varying degrees. While the exact prevalence of sexual impairments for CP/CPPS is not known, studies have consistently shown that erectile dysfunction, premature ejaculation, and painful ejaculation play a significant role in the overall quality of life in these patients. As such, the consideration of sexual dysfunction is a crucial part of the assessment when developing a treatment plan for patients.

12.2 Hypogonadism and Prostatitis

The association of prostatitis with endocrine disruption has been reported in literature dating back almost four decades. In 1978, Yunda et al. concluded that the degree and form of prostatitis may play a role in testicular endocrine function after finding reduced urinary testosterone excretion in patients with chronic prostatitis compared to controls [1]. Today the exact prevalence of low testosterone in patients with chronic prostatitis/chronic pelvic pain syndrome (CP/CPPS) is unknown. While a relationship between low testosterone and CP/CPPS has long been recognized, a causality dilemma

J. Syed
Department of Urology, University of Florida, College of Medicine,
Gainesville, FL, USA

V. Mouraviev (✉)
Department of Urology, Global Robotics Institute, Florida Hospital/
Celebration Health, Celebration, Kissimmee, FL, USA
e-mail: Vladimir.Mouraviev@flhosp.org

© Springer International Publishing Switzerland 2016
T. Cai, T.E. Bjerklund Johansen (eds.), *Prostatitis and Its Management: Concepts and Recommendations for Clinical Practice*, DOI 10.1007/978-3-319-25175-2_12

Fig. 12.1 Endocrine abnormalities leading to prostatic inflammation (Adopted from Pontari et al. [2] and Meng et al. [4])

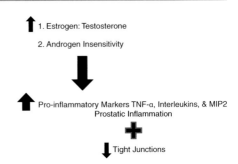

still remains. Leading theory, however, suggests that it is an initial increase in the estrogen-to-testosterone ratio that predisposes males to prostatitis (Fig. 12.1). This hypothesis is grounded on a variety of bench studies that have described the roles of these hormones on prostatic inflammation. Based on animal model predictions, estrogen likely plays a pro-inflammatory role by inducing the production of various cytokines such as TNF-α, MIP-2, and IL-6 [2]. On the other hand, testosterone has been shown to play an anti-inflammatory role by decreasing levels of cytokines such as TNF-α and MIP-1a [3]. Additionally, testosterone has recently been shown to play a role against inflammation by upregulating important proteins for tight junction ultrastructure; these tight junctions function as a barrier to infiltrating immune elements in the prostate gland [4]. Some patients may also experience a functional impairment of testosterone given certain genetic abnormalities. Men who are androgen insensitive will not benefit from the inflammatory protective features of testosterone and may be predisposed to prostatic inflammation.

12.3   Treatment of Low Testosterone in Patients with CP/ CPPS

Men with low testosterone may display symptoms of fatigue, sexual dysfunction, and decreased libido in addition to the common symptoms produced by CP/CPPS. These men will benefit from serum testosterone analysis and replacement therapy if a deficiency is found. While there is a paucity of literature on testosterone replacement therapy for hypogonadal patients with CP/CPPS, a recent study by Pang et al. has shown promising data [5]. Their study involved 48 patients, all of whom had a CP/CPPS history for at least 1 year, a score of at least 15 on the NIH-Chronic Prostatitis Symptom Index (NIH-CPSI), and a serum total testosterone concentration of less than 300 ng/dl [5]. Patients were treated with testosterone undecanoate 80 mg orally twice a day for 12 weeks [5]. After 12 weeks follow-up patients had significant improvements in NIH-CPSI totals and testosterone levels. Patients also experienced a benefit in terms of anxiety and depressive symptoms [5]. This initial study illustrates the various symptomatic benefits testosterone replacement therapy may offer to hypogonadal patients with CP/CPPS.

12.4   Sexual Dysfunction

Sexual dysfunction as a sequela of prostatitis is an umbrella term which encompasses a number of impairments. This includes erectile dysfunction (ED), premature ejaculation (PE), and painful ejaculation. Whether symptoms are actually caused by a primary or secondary process is still up for debate. Some argue that the urinary symptoms experienced by patients and the resultant impact on quality of life contribute to the sexual dysfunction seen. Nonetheless, there is a growing body of evidence on the prevalence of sexual dysfunction in patients with CP/CPPS. A study done in Turkey of 96 patients with microscopic evidence of prostatic inflammation revealed sexual dysfunction in 84 % of patients [6]. In a study done in China of 1786 men with chronic prostatitis, the overall prevalence of sexual dysfunction was found to be 49 %, with 7.7 % having both premature ejaculation and erectile dysfunction [7]. In another study from Turkey, 15.2 % of patients were found to have premature ejaculation and erectile dysfunction together [8]. Men who report both ED and ejaculatory difficulty also experience worse NIH-Chronic Prostatitis Symptom Index scores [9, 10]. It is important to note that when discussing the prevalence of the various sexual dysfunctions experienced by men with CP/CPPS, the statistics provided must be taken with a grain of salt. It has been recognized that the vast majority of evidence is based on questionnaire studies. This may limit the generalizability to practice; nonetheless the evidence is still compelling and can illuminate likely trends [11].

12.5   Erectile Dysfunction

Erectile dysfunction is defined as the consistent inability to achieve or maintain an erection for successful intercourse. Investigations on the prevalence of ED in men with CP/CPPS have reported varying numbers. One Chinese study estimated that the prevalence of ED in patients as assessed by the International Index of Erectile Function (IIEF-5) was 35.1 % [12]. A study performed in Italy of 399 men with symptoms of CP/CPPS found ED in 34 % [10]. A study of 296 patients in Malaysia found a component of ED either as a single symptom or in combination with ejaculatory dysfunction in 67 % of their study population [9]. A link between ED and a previous diagnosis of CP/CPPS has also been found. One case-control study reported that men with ED were more than three times more likely to have had previous CP/CPPS [13]. In terms of describing the underlying mechanism of ED in men with CP/CPPS, the research is scarce. There are, however, a few leading theories that should be discussed. Firstly, some patients may experience ED secondary to a low androgen status. Testosterone is hypothesized to exert its action on erectile function through peripheral and central mechanisms [14]. The frequency of sexual dysfunction increases as serum testosterone decreases and especially occurs with concentrations less than 225 ng/dl [10]. Other theories point to a vascular cause of ED. Prostatic inflammation may impair smooth muscle relaxation and vascularization of the prostate leading to suboptimal penile engorgement [13]. Additionally, it has been shown that men with CP/CPPS may have increased arterial stiffness resulting in a decreased filling of penile tissue with blood [15]. Afferent arterioles may also be externally compressed secondary to pelvic floor spasm exacerbating symptoms of ED [16]. Finally, there is an established association of CP/CPPS with psychogenic stress. Mood alterations secondary to pain and voiding dysfunction tend to reduce the frequency of sexual intercourse and contribute to a functional rather than an organic cause of ED. Any one of these mechanisms may contribute to ED in this patient population; however, a combination of physical and psychologic stress is likely responsible. The biologic rationale supported with the evidence of a high prevalence suggests that screening for ED among individuals with CP/CPPS is warranted.

12.6   Premature Ejaculation (PE)

PE is a poorly understood form of sexual dysfunction that is found to be commonly experienced by many healthy men. The definition has been established to encompass three main scenarios: ejaculation which occurs in a short time of vaginal penetration, usually within 1–3 min, the inability to delay ejaculation on nearly all vaginal penetrations, or a latency time that causes negative personal consequences such as distress or the avoidance of sexual intimacy in either the patient or partner. In line with the normal population of men, the actual prevalence of PE in men with CP/CPPS has not been established. There have, however, been a number of estimates cited in literature. One study from Turkey of 66 patients with CP/CPPS reported a 77.3 % PE rate [8]. An Italian study found a prevalence of premature ejaculation in their patient group to be 61.5 % [17]. A Chinese study of 600 men with CP/CPPS reported a PE prevalence of 30 % [18]. The differences in ethnicities and cultural attitudes toward sex may be an explanation for the spread of prevalence rates reported by these studies. Nonetheless, patients should be screened for symptoms of PE as the correlation with CP/CPPS has been consistently demonstrated. While the mechanism underlying the association of PE with CP/CPPS has not been clearly defined, two theories may explain the link. The first is the concept that prostatic inflammation alters sensation and the ejaculatory reflex. The resultant impairment of sensory feedback occurs prior to orgasm and may explain the mechanism of PE seen in patients with CP/CPPS [17]. A second theory is that patients with CP/CPPS may experience a significant amount of stress, depression, or anxiety. As a result of these psychologic factors, PE may develop. Ultimately, it is likely a combination of both biologic and social stressors plays a role in the development of PE.

12.7   Painful Ejaculation

Painful ejaculation is a pelviperineal pain caused by ejaculation or orgasm, and its prevalence rate is varied between 1 and 4 % in the general population [19]. Painful ejaculation is frequently seen in patients with CP/CPPS and has its own question within the NIH-CPSI [19]. The prevalence of painful ejaculation in CP/CPPS patients may range from 38 to 54 % based on reports from different studies [6, 9]. Men with painful ejaculation are more likely to be afflicted with additional symptoms. One multicenter study of 3700 patients found that of patients with painful ejaculation, 72 % also experienced erectile dysfunction. CP/CPPS patients with painful ejaculation also reported worse NIH-CPSI and quality of life scores [20]. The pathophysiologic explanation of painful ejaculation in patients with CP/CPPS is largely based on the inflammatory milieu seen in the prostate of these patients. With ejaculation, the contraction of an inflamed and irritated prostate gland can lead to severe pain and in many instances cause the patient to abstain from sexual activities [19].

12.8   Treatment of Sexual Dysfunction in Prostatitis

Therapeutic options that have been studied for the treatment of sexual dysfunction in men with CP/CPPS include alpha-adrenergic blockers and phosphodiesterase-5 (PDE5) inhibitors. Alpha-adrenergic inhibitors are thought to benefit sexual dysfunction symptoms through an indirect mechanism. By relaxing prostatic smooth muscle, men primarily experience improvements in lower urinary tract symptoms and as a result may report enhancement of sexual function. Alfuzosin 10 mg daily in men with painful ejaculation and lower urinary tract symptoms significantly improved urinary symptoms and ejaculatory and erectile dysfunction after 6 months of treatment [21]. PDE5 inhibitors may exhibit an impact in men with prostatitis by relaxing smooth muscle of prostatic ducts. This results in the washout of irritative inflammatory components in the prostatic tissue and may improve sexual symptoms [22]. One randomized study reported that mirodenafil 50 mg daily significantly improved IPSS, NIH-CPSI, and IIEF scores in men with CP/CPPS after 6 weeks of treatment [23]. The use of a combination therapy with alpha-blockers and PDE5 has not been shown to offer a statistically significant benefit in treating sexual symptoms of CP/CPPS over single therapy. In young CP/CPPS patients with ED, dual therapy with tamsulosin 4 mg daily plus sildenafil 50 mg used as necessary did not show a benefit in symptom scores when compared to tamsulosin monotherapy. Both groups did however report significant improvements in IPSS, NIH-CPSI, and IIEF scores when compared to baseline [24]. As the data is still evolving, there is no consensus on what the best therapy is for treating sexual dysfunction in men with CP/CPPS. The highest chance for success will likely involve approaching patients in a personalized manner and tackling each of their symptoms individually.

12.9   Summary

Andrologic sequelae in patients with prostatitis may include decreased testosterone, erectile dysfunction, painful ejaculation, and premature ejaculation. The prevalence of these symptoms in patients with CP/CPPS is high and plays a significant role in the morbidity of patients. A sexual function assessment is an important part of evaluating any patient with pelvic or perineal pain. Treatment strategies that have addressed sexual dysfunction include testosterone replacement therapy, alpha-adrenergic blockers, and PDE5s. Ultimately, treatment hinges on the prominent features of each individual's symptoms and requires a personalized approach.

References

1. Yunda IF, Imshinetskaya LP (1977) Testosterone excretion in chronic prostatitis. Andrologia 9:89–94
2. Pontari MA, Ruggieri MR (2004) Mechanisms in prostatitis/chronic pelvic pain syndrome. J Urol 172:839–845
3. Jia Y, Liu X, Yan J et al (2015) The alteration of inflammatory markers and apoptosis on chronic prostatitis induced by estrogen and androgen. Int Urol Nephrol 47:39–46
4. Meng J, Mostaghel EA, Vakar-Lopez F et al (2011) Testosterone regulates tight junction proteins and influences prostatic autoimmune responses. Horm Cancer 2:145–156
5. Pang R, Lu J, Zhou X et al (2015) MP25-02 testosterone replacement therapy for hypogonadal patients with chronic prostatitis/chronic pelvic pain syndrome. J Urol 193, e285
6. Tuncel A, Akbulut Z, Atan A et al (2006) Common symptoms in men with prostatic inflammation. Int Urol Nephrol 38:583–586
7. Liang C-Z, Zhang X-J, Hao Z-Y et al (2004) Prevalence of sexual dysfunction in Chinese men with chronic prostatitis. BJU Int 93:568–570
8. Gonen M, Kalkan M, Cenker A et al (2005) Prevalence of premature ejaculation in Turkish men with chronic pelvic pain syndrome. J Androl 26:601–603
9. Lee SWH, Liong ML, Yuen KH et al (2008) Adverse impact of sexual dysfunction in chronic prostatitis/chronic pelvic pain syndrome. Urology 71:79–84
10. Trinchieri A, Magri V, Cariani L et al (2007) Prevalence of sexual dysfunction in men with chronic prostatitis/chronic pelvic pain syndrome. Arch Ital Urol Androl Organo Uff Soc Ital Ecogr Urol E Nefrol Assoc Ric Urol 79:67–70
11. Shoskes DA (2012) The challenge of erectile dysfunction in the man with chronic prostatitis/chronic pelvic pain syndrome. Curr Urol Rep 13:263–267
12. Hao Z-Y, Li H-J, Wang Z-P et al (2011) The prevalence of erectile dysfunction and its relation to chronic prostatitis in Chinese men. J Androl 32:496–501
13. Chung S-D, Keller JJ, Lin H-C (2012) A case-control study on the association between chronic prostatitis/chronic pelvic pain syndrome and erectile dysfunction. BJU Int 110:726–730
14. Guay AT (2006) Testosterone and erectile physiology. Aging Male: Off J Int Soc Study Aging Male 9:201–206
15. Shoskes DA, Prots D, Karns J et al (2011) Greater endothelial dysfunction and arterial stiffness in men with chronic prostatitis/chronic pelvic pain syndrome--a possible link to cardiovascular disease. J Urol 186:907–910
16. Shoskes DA, Berger R, Elmi A et al (2008) Muscle tenderness in men with chronic prostatitis/chronic pelvic pain syndrome: the chronic prostatitis cohort study. J Urol 179:556–560
17. Screponi E, Carosa E, Di Stasi SM et al (2001) Prevalence of chronic prostatitis in men with premature ejaculation. Urology 58:198–202
18. Mo M-Q, Long L-L, Xie W-L et al (2014) Sexual dysfunctions and psychological disorders associated with type IIIa chronic prostatitis: a clinical survey in China. Int Urol Nephrol 46:2255–2261
19. Delavierre D, Sibert L, Rigaud J et al (2014) Painful ejaculation. Prog En Urol J Assoc Fr Urol Société Fr Urol 24:414–420
20. Tran CN, Shoskes DA (2013) Sexual dysfunction in chronic prostatitis/chronic pelvic pain syndrome. World J Urol 31:741–746

21. Nickel JC, Elhilali M, Emberton M et al (2006) The beneficial effect of alfuzosin 10 mg once daily in "real-life" practice on lower urinary tract symptoms (LUTS), quality of life and sexual dysfunction in men with LUTS and painful ejaculation. BJU Int 97:1242–1246
22. Grimsley SJS, Khan MH, Jones GE (2007) Mechanism of phosphodiesterase 5 inhibitor relief of prostatitis symptoms. Med Hypotheses 69:25–26
23. Kong DH, Yun CJ, Park HJ et al (2014) The efficacy of mirodenafil for chronic prostatitis/chronic pelvic pain syndrome in middle-aged males. World J Mens Health 32:145–150
24. Cantoro U, Catanzariti F, Lacetera V et al (2013) Comparison of tamsulosin vs tamsulosin/sildenafil effectiveness in the treatment of erectile dysfunction in patients affected by type III chronic prostatitis. Arch Ital Urol Androl Organo Uff Soc Ital Ecogr Urol E Nefrol Assoc Ric Urol 85:109–112

The Role of Chronic Prostatitis in Male Infertility: Is There a Relationship?

13

Vitaly Smelov

13.1 Introduction

13.1.1 Infertility and Prostatitis

The World Health Organization (WHO) classifies infertility as "a disease of the reproductive system defined by the failure to achieve a clinical pregnancy after 12 months or more of regular unprotected sexual intercourse" [102]. In fact, the period when practicing regular unprotected sex might result in pregnancy varies from the first 3 months in 20–37 % of the couples younger than age 30 [76] till up to 3 years in 93 % for every 100 couples from the general population [66]. Depending on the definition used, the prevalence estimates across populations vary widely between 3.3 % and 26.4 % for current infertility and between 2.6 % and 31.8 % for lifetime infertility, respectively [34]. Studies suggest that about 15% and 10% of couples, who have not achieved pregnancy within 1 and 2 years, seek a medical treatment for infertility [33, 54, 76]. Current general understanding is that for couples, who have been trying to conceive for more than 3 years without success, the likelihood of pregnancy occurring within the next year is 25 % or less [66].

Importantly, while a common belief is that infertility remains a "women's problem," it is a couple-based clinical problem. In fact, male factors have been accepted for approximately 20 % of couple infertility with another 30–40 % presenting with reproductive abnormalities in both partners [4, 91].

V. Smelov
Screening Group, International Agency for Research on Cancer, World Health Organization, Lyon, France

Department of Urology and Andrology, North-Western State Medical University named after I.I. Mechnikov, St. Petersburg, Russia
e-mail: vitsmelov@yahoo.com

© Springer International Publishing Switzerland 2016
T. Cai, T.E. Bjerklund Johansen (eds.), *Prostatitis and Its Management: Concepts and Recommendations for Clinical Practice*, DOI 10.1007/978-3-319-25175-2_13

117

Multiple factors can lead to reduced male fertility. In about 50 % of cases, the cause of male infertility cannot be determined [40]. Among the known [97] categories, 6,6–12 % of accepted causes are due to urogenital tract infections [21, 94, 97]. It is unknown how many of these cases are caused by prostatitis (inflammation of the prostate gland). The prostate disorder is listed by the WHO among male accessory genital gland infections [97] and is one of the most common urological problems affecting men in their reproductive age, accounting for 8 % of all urologist visits [15] and an overall lifetime prevalence of 14 % [63]. Recent discoveries on the prostate and its function provide new insight to the magnitude of the problem.

13.1.2 Prostate Gland and Prostatic Secretion

The prostate is the largest male accessory genital gland. The normal prostate reaches 20 ± 6 g in men between 21 and 30 years old, and this weight remains essentially constant with increasing age unless benign prostatic hyperplasia develops [8]. The 25–30 prostate glandular units (acini) and their ducts, which enter the prostatic urethra, are lined with secretory epithelium and surrounded by a variable amount of stroma, housing different stromal cell types with distinct phenotypes [31, 61].

Prostate secretions represent the second portion of the ejaculate and contribute up to 30 % to the total volume of human semen, which is a mixture of components produced by several different glands and should exceed 1.5 mL, or even 2.5 mL, as the lower limit of normal semen volume [16, 72]. Notably, impaired sperm parameters in patients with prostate disorders have been shown in some studies [93]. The prostate gland has the highest concentration of zinc in the human body [12] and is rich with citric acid [43]. Decreased quantities of zinc, citric acid, phosphatase and fructose [95], alpha-glutamyl transferase activity [95], and, potentially, quantities of potassium, sodium, and calcium [101] can be considered as indicators of disturbed prostatic secretion.

The physical access to the prostate gland is limited, and current guidelines [9, 32] recommend the evaluation of expressed prostatic secretion (EPS) by microscopy and culture in patients with prostatitis-like symptoms or a prostate biopsy for confirming or ruling out malignancy when indicated. EPS can be obtained during digital rectal examination (DRE, a routine urological diagnostic procedure) with massage of the prostate. The investigation of EPS has been commonly used in urology ever since the Meares-Stamey 4-glass test was described. The test includes a quantitative culture of pure EPS and was launched in 1968 [62] and became the gold standard for assessing the bacteriological and inflammatory state of the lower urinary tract in urological patients. The test has later been replaced by an easier-to-perform two-glass or pre-post-massage screening test [67, 68]. Since infections of the prostate impair the gland's excretory function, the investigation of EPS is currently recommended in clinical routine assessment of non-acute conditions [32].

13.1.3 Classification of Prostatitis

The predominant symptoms of prostatitis are pain at various locations and lower urinary tract symptoms [2, 3, 103]. In fact, the term "prostatitis" has included bacterial prostatitis, with a detected infective agent, and the term "prostatitis syndrome" or chronic pelvic pain syndrome (CPPS), when no infective agent is found and which is presumably of multifactorial origin [32].

The currently recommended [32] classification distinguishes prostatitis from CPPS and employs such criteria as the duration of symptoms (classified as chronic, if they persist for at least 3 months) and evidence of inflammation and infection [62] localized to the prostate. It was suggested by the US National Institute of Diabetes and Digestive and Kidney Diseases (NIDDK) of the National Institutes of Health (NIH) and includes four types of prostatitis: acute (type I) and chronic (type II) bacterial prostatitis; chronic abacterial prostatitis or CPPS (type III), with inflammatory (IIIA) and noninflammatory subtypes (IIIB); and asymptomatic inflammatory prostatitis (type IV) [44, 51, 79].

13.1.3.1 Acute Bacterial Prostatitis

Ascending urethral infection, the reflux of infected urine into the prostate, or the lower urinary tract manipulations might result in developing acute bacterial prostatitis (ABP). It is a life-threatening infection with fever, nausea, intense perineal or suprapubic pain, and voiding symptoms, which might culminate in urosepsis or the development of prostatic abscess. In this situation, prostatic massage is contraindicated, and the most important bacteriological investigation of the patient is the midstream urine culture. Among the most common causative organisms are gram-negative urinary pathogens, such as *E. coli*, followed by *Klebsiella, Proteus, Pseudomonas*, and *Enterococcus* [26]. An additional group of microorganisms of debatable significance includes staphylococci, streptococci, *Corynebacterium* sp., *Chlamydia trachomatis, Ureaplasma urealyticum*, and *Mycoplasma hominis* [83, 96]. Acute prostatitis usually requires parenteral treatment with bactericidal antibiotics of high doses [32]. Although current data provides no evidence for the direct impact of this condition on male infertility, the latter can be affected through the complications of ABP, such as epididymitis and chronic prostatitis. It has been reported that chronic infection, predominantly chronic bacterial prostatitis or epididymo-orchitis, and inflammatory chronic pelvic pain syndrome are the outcomes of acute bacterial prostatitis in 10.2 % and 9.6 % of patients, respectively [100].

13.1.3.2 Chronic Bacterial Prostatitis

Chronic bacterial prostatitis (CBP) has been considered as a relatively rare clinical condition, since a causative pathogen is detected by routine methods in only 5–10 % of cases [96]. The current clinical definition of bacterial prostatitis describes it as "a disease entity diagnosed clinically and by evidence of inflammation and infection localized to the prostate" [32]. The most common pathogens in CBP are similar to the ones detected in ABP [32].

A better understanding of the direct impact of pathogens is necessary to shed light on the significance of CBP for the development of male infertility. In fact, the prevalence of different bacterial species in male populations – and their relevance to the etiology of male infertility – varies according to geographical distribution [70]. It has been speculated that, due to an impairment of the secretory capacity of the prostate, proven bacterial infections of the male reproductive tract might impact negatively on all parameters evaluated in semen [22, 56].

Most of the studies have been done with *Escherichia coli*. The pathogen is usually cultured from bladder urine during infectious episodes but not at other times [81] and has been considered to be responsible for the great majority of cases of CBP [96]. It has been reported that infection with *E. coli* results in mitochondrial changes and membrane alterations in sperm cells [29], decreased percentage of sperm with intact mitochondrial membrane potential [84], immobilization, and impaired acrosomal function in human spermatozoa [18], that finally causes the decrease of sperm viability and motility [56, 84]. Observational studies on the significance of positive bacterial semen cultures have speculated a potential harm of *Enterococcus, S. epidermidis, S. aureus, P. aeruginosa*, and *Klebsiella* on male fertility [7, 27, 56, 71]. In addition to obtaining relief of clinical symptoms, all the effects on fertility provide a rationale [32] for start of antibacterial treatment.

Chlamydia trachomatis
Another intensively studied pathogen is *C. trachomatis*. Chlamydia is the most commonly detected bacterial sexually transmitted infection (STI) worldwide, and the numbers of infections keep increasing [13, 23, 98]. Mostly asymptomatic [14], chlamydia infection is a major cause of infertility [98], mostly among females. Although no significant differences between infertile and fertile men in terms of the prevalence of *C. trachomatis* have been reported [52], large epidemiological data suggest an association of a past *C. trachomatis* infection with infertility in men [41]. Chlamydia has been directly associated with decreased sperm motility as well as abnormal sperm concentration and morphology [10, 24]. The pathogen has been reported to be able to attach to human spermatozoa, which results in their *C. trachomatis*-induced death in vitro [38]. Albeit the proven biological significance of chlamydia infection in male infertility has only been accepted for acute epididymitis and subsequent azoospermia [78], the pathogen has been associated with decreased sperm motility and abnormal sperm concentration and morphology in young prostatitis patients [59].

Nevertheless, the role of chlamydia infection in the pathogenesis of prostatitis remains inconclusive and controversial. *C. trachomatis* has been detected in semen samples of male partners in infertile couples [50], in the fluid of dilated seminal vesicles [30] and EPS [87], and in prostate tissue removed by transurethral resection or by open surgery [17], or obtained via perineal approach [45], but the discrimination from possible urethral contamination of the obtained material remains impossible to exclude.

Interestingly, chlamydia infection has been associated with increased leukocyte counts and pain severity in men with CPPS [73], and the role of immune system activation in the pathophysiology of chronic prostatitis has been proposed [60].

Some studies suggested anti-*C. trachomatis* immunoglobulin A (IgA) as a more sensitive marker for detection of *C. trachomatis* prostatitis than currently used amplification or culture techniques. Interestingly, a significant increase in mucosal IgA has been detected in the ejaculate of men with chronic prostatitis as compared to controls, and, also, significant correlations between IL-8 and mucosal IgA and between IL-8 levels and prostate symptom score results were found [59, 60].

Genital Mycoplasmas

Among genital mycoplasmas, *Mycoplasma genitalium* has also been considered as an STI [77]. However, their role in chronic prostatitis and related male subfertility is even more controversial that in the case of chlamydia infection. In fact, *M. genitalium* has been detected by amplification techniques in semen from some men with chronic abacterial inflammatory prostatitis [55] and, also, in a small number of prostatic biopsy specimens [46]. On the other hand, an earlier study failed to detect mycoplasmas in all biopsy specimens [20].

No significant differences have been reported between infertile and fertile men in terms of the prevalence of *U. urealyticum* and *M. hominis* [52]. Importantly, being untreated or successfully treated, the ascending urethral infection caused by genital mycoplasmas might trigger the immune response that would involve the prostate. In fact, an early infection might set in motion immunological processes that culminate in chronic prostatitis [90], which may potentially affect male fertility.

Novel Diagnostic Approaches Are Changing the Routine

Further studies, employing novel diagnostic approaches, are required to investigate the clinical significance of the infective pathogens and potential mechanisms of action in male infertility. Culture tests and microscopy have been considered as the gold standard for diagnosing urinary tract infections (UTIs), with an additional amplification system used if sexually transmitted pathogens are suspected [32, 51]. However, the current evaluation of UTIs, under the umbrella of "significant bacteriuria" first introduced in 1960 [42], was based on analyses of a cultured single bacterial isolate assembly representing the dominant pathogen. A significant limitation in the current widely used method is the detection of only culturable bacteria. The method is also limited in the detection of multiple pathogens or the strain diversity. Thus, caution is required when considering studied human-ejaculated sperm or EPS as "sterile" based on the lack of bacteria detected by classical methods alone. The wide use of amplification methods in detection of urogenital pathogens, in particular STIs [23], is a result of the methods' good specificity and sufficient sensitivity. Noteworthily, only good laboratory practice and monitoring reference reagents should be employed [92], to be able to differentiate between infection and contamination. These detection methods are rapid and some of them allow detection of several pathogens during the same experiment. For instance, a novel bead-based multiplex assay is using a multiplex PCR followed by Luminex bead-based hybridization and has shown its effectiveness in assessing 18 urogenital infections in the same experiment [82]. However, the abovementioned tests are able to detect already known pathogens. The novel metagenomic sequencing (MGS) approach allows comprehensive high-throughput analyses in a sample without prior cloning, and it has become instrumental in detecting a broad range of non-culturable bacteria in "sterile" (based on "classical" diagnostic practices) EPS. The recent first-in-principle study on MGS of EPS found several bacterial reads in men with chronic prostatic inflammation. Most of the obtained bacterial sequences belonged to the family Proteobacteria, which includes such main causative agents of bacterial prostatitis as *E. coli*, *Klebsiella*, *Shigella*, *Proteus*, *Enterobacter*, etc. [86]. These findings raise the question of whether MGS could be useful for microbiological diagnosis in some cases, when conventional diagnostics may have failed to identify an appropriate treatment [6]. MGS studies would be also beneficial in exploring the prostate microbiome and in discovery of the role of potential non-culturable bacterial or viral cofactors in particular. For instance, in a population of prostatitis-related symptoms attributable to chlamydia infection, coinfection with human papillomavirus (HPV) was found to have a significant role in decreasing male fertility, in particular with regard to sperm motility and morphology [11]. A highly statistically significant correlation between pregnancy loss rate after the assisted reproductive technologies and positive HPV DNA testing in semen samples has been reported [75], providing an additional support that HPV coinfection may be related to impaired sperm motility [58], as well as other potential bacterial and viral coinfections. For cost reasons it will take time before novel assays become clinically applicable, but while the MGS methods remain expensive, the sequencing-related costs have decreased rapidly. This might significantly change the current viewpoint on the pathogenesis of prostatic disorders where bacteria may not play a role, such as chronic abacterial prostatitis.

13.1.3.3 Chronic Prostatitis/Chronic Pelvic Pain Syndrome (CP/CPPS)

The current culture- and microcopy-based diagnostic approach discriminates most cases of chronic prostatitis as abacterial or chronic pelvic pain syndrome (CPPS). The impact of chronic abacterial prostatitis on semen parameters remains controversial [36, 49, 53, 64, 74]. Interestingly, no difference was found in the sperm parameters between the two subcategories of CPPS (NIH CPPS IIIA versus IIIB) [36]. The exact etiology of CPPS is not completely understood, and several mechanisms have been speculated to affect the male fertility in the absence of the pathogen.

Prostate Ejaculatory and Secretory Dysfunctions

The reduced volume of EPS may result in decreased semen volume. This can be a result of both secretory and ejaculatory dysfunctions. The role of male sex gland infections in diminishing the volume of EPS was observed in 1999 [95], but the mechanism of dysfunction in prostatitis remains unclear. The prostate infection may decrease the production of enzymes or secretion of citric acid, alpha-glucosidase, fructose, and zinc [56] or increase semen viscosity [25, 48], which adversely affects sperm motility. A complete lack of sperm occurs in about 10–15 % of infertile men. In fact, the most common problems in such cases are related to the testicles, hormone imbalances, or blockages in the male reproductive organs. However, chronic prostatitis may result in premature ejaculation [104] and ejaculatory and erectile dysfunctions [48]. The lack of sexual desire can be an additional component of sexual dysfunctions. These situations may lead to a decreased number of sexual intercourses. In order to optimize the likelihood of conception, a frequency of sexual intercourse from 2 to 3 times weekly was recommended [89].

Inflammatory Mediators
Inflammation in the prostate gland has been speculated to promote an autoimmune response, which might be leading to deleterious effects on semen quality and function [28, 65]. Moreover, anti-inflammatory treatment has been reported to have a positive impact on sperm parameters [93], although the exact details remain unclear. The originally suggested [39] role of prostatitis-induced antisperm antibodies against human sperm has not been supported in later studies [37, 56]. Instead, poor semen quality has been linked with the potential role of multiple cytokines, such as seminal interleukins 6, 8, 10, 12, and 18 and TNF-alpha [57, 65], in which detection might also be dependent on the presence of leukocytes or bacterial pathogens [57]. Although the leukocyte (or white blood cell (WBC)) counts may not correlate with the severity of symptoms [80], they are known to produce seminal reactive oxygen species (ROS) in response to infection or inflammation stimuli [74]. An abnormal ROS level is associated with human infertility in several ways, including some STIs, in particular *C. trachomatis* [10]. Increased levels of ROS are associated with leukocytospermia [85] and may lead to damage of cell membranes, intracellular proteins, organelles, [69] and sperm DNA [1, 69], with subsequent impairment of sperm motility [5] and decreased seminal total antioxidant capacity [74]. Interestingly, while increased seminal WBCs in the ejaculate of patients with CPPS were not found to affect semen parameters [53], elevated seminal leukocytes alone were associated with poor semen parameters [22]. An increased amount of ROS in semen is also linked to high DNA fragmentation index (DFI), a measure of the proportion of sperms with chromosome breaks and a predictor of male fertility independent of standard sperm parameters. Urogenital infections have been reported to imply increase in DFI [88]. However, although the role of oxidative stress has been associated with prostatitis and male infertility [47], the true pathways remain controversial, requiring further studies.

13.1.3.4 Asymptomatic Inflammatory Prostatitis
Asymptomatic inflammatory prostatitis (AIP) has been considered as a relatively rare disorder. However any prevalence data on AIP might be biased because of the nature of this prostate disorder: men with AIP present no symptoms, and, thus, the disorder is incidentally detected by prostatic biopsies to rule out prostate cancer or during an infertility workup [19]. The evidence of infections is based on the detection of increased number of leukocytes in prostate biopsy, seminal fluid, EPS, or voided bladder urine. The WHO defines leukocytospermia as the presence of $\geq 1 \times 10^6$ WBC/ml [99]. In prostatic fluid, 5–15 WBCs per high power field are generally considered as abnormal [80]. Studies on the potential role of AIP in male infertility are very limited. One retrospective study reported that a 3-week course of empirical antibiotic therapy applied to the male partners of infertile couples resolves

leukocytospermia and improves the natural pregnancy rate among infertile couples, suggesting that low-level leukocytospermia has deleterious effects on male fertility [35]. AIP should be distinguished from CBP and CPPS.

Conclusions

The prostate gland plays an important role in the production of seminal fluid and the delivery of sperm during male ejaculation. Prostate infection and inflammation may affect the male fertility, and chronic prostatitis has been recognized as one of the causes of male infertility. However, several speculated pathways are poorly understood, and there is no general consensus on the exact mechanisms of prostatitis-induced infertility. In fact, while the vast majority of chronic prostatitis has been considered as abacterial, novel diagnostic approaches as MGS and some others are close to change this paradigm by discovering non-culturable microorganisms in men with chronic prostate disorders. These discoveries on prostate microbiome will help to determine the role of pathogens as potential cofactors in prostatitis-related infertility. Importantly, chronic prostatitis is a long-lasting, often recurrent, disorder with controversial evidence of infections in a gland with limited physical access. Future studies should also focus on the importance of prostate cellular and humoral anti-inflammatory response for male fertility, with contemporary biomarkers.

Take-Home Message
- Infertility workup should include the evaluation of prostate infection and inflammation.
- The impact of chronic prostatitis on semen parameters remains controversial.
- Current detection methods do not detect non-culturable pathogens.
- Further research on the role of prostate microbiome and inflammatory markers is warranted.

References

1. Aitken RJ, Krausz C (2001) Oxidative stress, DNA damage and the Y chromosome. Reprod Camb Engl 122:497–506
2. Alexander RB, Ponniah S, Hasday J, Hebel JR (1998) Elevated levels of proinflammatory cytokines in the semen of patients with chronic prostatitis/chronic pelvic pain syndrome. Urology 52:744–749
3. Alexander RB, Trissel D (1996) Chronic prostatitis: results of an Internet survey. Urology 48:568–574
4. Anderson JE, Farr SL, Jamieson DJ, Warner L, Macaluso M (2009) Infertility services reported by men in the United States: national survey data. Fertil Steril 91:2466–2470. doi:10.1016/j.fertnstert.2008.03.022
5. Armstrong JS, Rajasekaran M, Chamulitrat W, Gatti P, Hellstrom WJ, Sikka SC (1999) Characterization of reactive oxygen species induced effects on human spermatozoa movement and energy metabolism. Free Radic Biol Med 26:869–880

6. Becla L, Lunshof JE, Gurwitz D, In S, den Bäumen T, Westerhoff HV, Lange BMH, Brand A (2011) Health technology assessment in the era of personalized health care. Int J Technol Assess Health Care 27:118–126. doi:10.1017/S026646231100002X

7. Berktas M, Aydin S, Yilmaz Y, Cecen K, Bozkurt H (2008) Sperm motility changes after coincubation with various uropathogenic microorganisms: an in vitro experimental study. Int Urol Nephrol 40:383–389. doi:10.1007/s11255-007-9289-4

8. Berry SJ, Coffey DS, Walsh PC, Ewing LL (1984) The development of human benign prostatic hyperplasia with age. J Urol 132:474–479

9. Bolla M, van Casteren NJ, Cornford P, Culine S, Joniau S, Lam T, Mason MD, Matveev V, van der Poel H, van der Kwast TH, others (2015) Guidelines on prostate cancer. EAU Guidelines. European Association of Urology, In

10. Boncompain G, Schneider B, Delevoye C, Kellermann O, Dautry-Varsat A, Subtil A (2010) Production of reactive oxygen species is turned on and rapidly shut down in epithelial cells infected with Chlamydia trachomatis. Infect Immun 78:80–87. doi:10.1128/IAI.00725-09

11. Cai T, Wagenlehner FME, Mondaini N, D' EC, Meacci F, Migno S, Malossini G, Mazzoli S, Bartoletti R (2014) Effect of human papillomavirus and Chlamydia trachomatis co-infection on sperm quality in young heterosexual men with chronic prostatitis-related symptoms. BJU Int 113:281–287. doi:10.1111/bju.12244

12. Caldamone AA, Freytag MK, Cockett AT (1979) Seminal zinc and male infertility. Urology 13:280–281

13. CDC (2014) Centers for Disease Control and Prevention. Chlamydia – CDC fact sheet. http://www.cdc.gov/std/chlamydia/stdfact-chlamydia.htm. Accessed 8 Jul 2015

14. Clarivet B, Picot E, Marchandin H, Tribout V, Rachedi N, Schwartzentruber E, Ledésert B, Dereure O, Guillot B, Picot M-C (2014) Prevalence of Chlamydia trachomatis, Neisseria gonorrhoeae and Mycoplasma genitalium in asymptomatic patients under 30 years of age screened in a French sexually transmitted infections clinic. Eur J Dermatol EJD 24:611–616. doi:10.1684/ejd.2014.2413

15. Collins MM, Stafford RS, O'Leary MP, Barry MJ (1998) How common is prostatitis? A national survey of physician visits. J Urol 159:1224–1228

16. Cooper TG, Noonan E, von Eckardstein S, Auger J, Baker HWG, Behre HM, Haugen TB, Kruger T, Wang C, Mbizvo MT, Vogelsong KM (2010) World Health Organization reference values for human semen characteristics. Hum Reprod Update 16:231–245. doi:10.1093/humupd/dmp048

17. Corradi G, Bucsek M, Pánovics J, Verebélyi A, Kardos M, Kádár A, Frang D (1996) Detection of Chlamydia trachomatis in the prostate by in-situ hybridization and by transmission electron microscopy. Int J Androl 19:109–112

18. Diemer T, Huwe P, Michelmann HW, Mayer F, Schiefer HG, Weidner W (2000) Escherichia coli-induced alterations of human spermatozoa. An electron microscopy analysis. Int J Androl 23:178–186

19. Dimitrakov J, Diemer T, Ludwig M, Weidner W (2001) Recent developments in diagnosis and therapy of the prostatitis syndromes. Curr Opin Urol 11:87–91

20. Doble A, Thomas BJ, Furr PM, Walker MM, Harris JR, Witherow RO, Taylor-Robinson D (1989) A search for infectious agents in chronic abacterial prostatitis using ultrasound guided biopsy. Br J Urol 64:297–301

21. Dohle GR (2003) Inflammatory-associated obstructions of the male reproductive tract. Andrologia 35:321–324

22. Domes T, Lo KC, Grober ED, Mullen JBM, Mazzulli T, Jarvi K (2012) The incidence and effect of bacteriospermia and elevated seminal leukocytes on semen parameters. Fertil Steril 97:1050–1055. doi:10.1016/j.fertnstert.2012.01.124

23. ECDC (2015) European Centre for Disease Prevention and Control. Chlamydia. c2005-2015. http://ecdc.europa.eu/en/healthtopics/chlamydia/Pages/index.aspx. Accessed 8 Jul 2015

24. Eley A, Pacey AA, Galdiero M, Galdiero M, Galdiero F (2005) Can Chlamydia trachomatis directly damage your sperm? Lancet Infect Dis 5:53–57. doi:10.1016/S1473-3099(04)01254-X

25. Elia J, Delfino M, Imbrogno N, Capogreco F, Lucarelli M, Rossi T, Mazzilli F (2009) Human semen hyperviscosity: prevalence, pathogenesis and therapeutic aspects. Asian J Androl 11:609–615. doi:10.1038/aja.2009.46

26. Etienne M, Chavanet P, Sibert L, Michel F, Levesque H, Lorcerie B, Doucet J, Pfitzenmeyer P, Caron F (2008) Acute bacterial prostatitis: heterogeneity in diagnostic criteria and management. Retrospective multicentric analysis of 371 patients diagnosed with acute prostatitis. BMC Infect Dis 8:12. doi:10.1186/1471-2334-8-12

27. Filipiak E, Marchlewska K, Oszukowska E, Walczak-Jedrzejowska R, Swierczynska-Cieplucha A, Kula K, Slowikowska-Hilczer J (2014) Presence of aerobic micro-organisms and their influence on basic semen parameters in infertile men. Andrologia. doi:10.1111/and.12338

28. Fraczek M, Kurpisz M (2007) Inflammatory mediators exert toxic effects of oxidative stress on human spermatozoa. J Androl 28:325–333. doi:10.2164/jandrol.106.001149

29. Fraczek M, Piasecka M, Gaczarzewicz D, Szumala-Kakol A, Kazienko A, Lenart S, Laszczynska M, Kurpisz M (2012) Membrane stability and mitochondrial activity of human-ejaculated spermatozoa during in vitro experimental infection with Escherichia coli, Staphylococcus haemolyticus and Bacteroides ureolyticus. Andrologia 44:315–329. doi:10.1111/j.1439-0272.2012.01283.x

30. Furuya R, Takahashi S, Furuya S, Kunishima Y, Takeyama K, Tsukamoto T (2004) Is seminal vesiculitis a discrete disease entity? Clinical and microbiological study of seminal vesiculitis in patients with acute epididymitis. J Urol 171:1550–1553. doi:10.1097/01.ju.0000116288.59223.e9

31. Gevaert T, Lerut E, Joniau S, Franken J, Roskams T, De Ridder D (2014) Characterization of subepithelial interstitial cells in normal and pathological human prostate. Histopathology 65:418–428. doi:10.1111/his.12402

32. Grabe M, Bartoletti R, Bjerklund Johansen TE, Cai T, Çek M, Köves B, Naber KG, Pickard RS, Tenke P, Wagenlehner F, Wullt B (2015) EAU Guidelines on Urological Infections. EAU Guidelines. European Association of Urology, In

33. Greenhall E, Vessey M (1990) The prevalence of subfertility: a review of the current confusion and a report of two new studies. Fertil Steril 54:978–983

34. Gurunath S, Pandian Z, Anderson RA, Bhattacharya S (2011) Defining infertility – a systematic review of prevalence studies. Hum Reprod Update 17:575–588. doi:10.1093/humupd/dmr015

35. Hamada A, Agarwal A, Sharma R, French DB, Ragheb A, Sabanegh ES (2011) Empirical treatment of low-level leukocytospermia with doxycycline in male infertility patients. Urology 78:1320–1325. doi:10.1016/j.urology.2011.08.062

36. Henkel R, Ludwig M, Schuppe H-C, Diemer T, Schill W-B, Weidner W (2006) Chronic pelvic pain syndrome/chronic prostatitis affect the acrosome reaction in human spermatozoa. World J Urol 24:39–44. doi:10.1007/s00345-005-0038-y

37. Hoover P, Naz RK (2012) Do men with prostate abnormalities (prostatitis/benign prostatic hyperplasia/prostate cancer) develop immunity to spermatozoa or seminal plasma? Int J Androl 35:608–615. doi:10.1111/j.1365-2605.2011.01246.x

38. Hosseinzadeh S, Pacey AA, Eley A (2003) Chlamydia trachomatis-induced death of human spermatozoa is caused primarily by lipopolysaccharide. J Med Microbiol 52:193–200

39. Jarow JP, Kirkland JA, Assimos DG (1990) Association of antisperm antibodies with chronic nonbacterial prostatitis. Urology 36:154–156

40. Jose-Miller AB, Boyden JW, Frey KA (2007) Infertility. Am Fam Physician 75:849–856

41. Karinen L, Pouta A, Hartikainen AL, Bloigu A, Paldanius M, Leinonen M, Saikku P, Järvelin MR (2004) Association between Chlamydia trachomatis antibodies and subfertility in the Northern Finland Birth Cohort 1966 (NFBC 1966), at the age of 31 years. Epidemiol Infect 132:977–984

42. Kass EH (1960) Bacteriuria and pyelonephritis of pregnancy. Arch Intern Med 105:194–198

43. Kavanagh JP (1994) Isocitric and citric acid in human prostatic and seminal fluid: implications for prostatic metabolism and secretion. Prostate 24:139–142

44. Krieger JN, Nyberg L, Nickel JC (1999) NIH consensus definition and classification of prostatitis. JAMA 282:236–237
45. Krieger JN, Riley DE (2002) Prostatitis: what is the role of infection. Int J Antimicrob Agents 19:475–479
46. Krieger JN, Riley DE, Roberts MC, Berger RE (1996) Prokaryotic DNA sequences in patients with chronic idiopathic prostatitis. J Clin Microbiol 34:3120–3128
47. Kullisaar T, Türk S, Punab M, Mändar R (2012) Oxidative stress – cause or consequence of male genital tract disorders? Prostate 72:977–983. doi:10.1002/pros.21502
48. La Vignera S, Condorelli R, Vicari E, Agata RD', Calogero AE (2012) High frequency of sexual dysfunction in patients with male accessory gland infections. Andrologia 44(Suppl 1):438–446. doi:10.1111/j.1439-0272.2011.01202.x
49. Leib Z, Bartoov B, Eltes F, Servadio C (1994) Reduced semen quality caused by chronic abacterial prostatitis: an enigma or reality? Fertil Steril 61:1109–1116
50. Levy R, Layani-Milon MP, Giscard D'Estaing S, Najioullah F, Lornage J, Aymard M, Lina B (1999) Screening for Chlamydia trachomatis and Ureaplasma urealyticum infection in semen from asymptomatic male partners of infertile couples prior to in vitro fertilization. Int J Androl 22:113–118
51. Litwin MS, McNaughton-Collins M, Fowler FJ, Nickel JC, Calhoun EA, Pontari MA, Alexander RB, Farrar JT, O'Leary MP (1999) The National Institutes of Health chronic prostatitis symptom index: development and validation of a new outcome measure. Chronic Prostatitis Collaborative Research Network. J Urol 162:369–375
52. Liu J, Wang Q, Ji X, Guo S, Dai Y, Zhang Z, Jia L, Shi Y, Tai S, Lee Y (2014) Prevalence of Ureaplasma urealyticum, Mycoplasma hominis, Chlamydia trachomatis infections, and semen quality in infertile and fertile men in China. Urology 83:795–799. doi:10.1016/j.urology.2013.11.009
53. Ludwig M, Vidal A, Huwe P, Diemer T, Pabst W, Weidner W (2003) Significance of inflammation on standard semen analysis in chronic prostatitis/chronic pelvic pain syndrome. Andrologia 35:152–156
54. Male Infertility Best Practice Policy Committee of the American Urological Association, Practice Committee of the American Society for Reproductive Medicine (2006) Report on optimal evaluation of the infertile male. Fertil Steril 86:S202–S209. doi:10.1016/j.fertnstert.2006.08.029
55. Mändar R, Raukas E, Türk S, Korrovits P, Punab M (2005) Mycoplasmas in semen of chronic prostatitis patients. Scand J Urol Nephrol 39:479–482. doi:10.1080/00365590500199822
56. Marconi M, Pilatz A, Wagenlehner F, Diemer T, Weidner W (2009) Impact of infection on the secretory capacity of the male accessory glands. Int Braz J Urol Off J Braz Soc Urol 35:299–308; discussion 308–309
57. Martínez-Prado E, Camejo Bermúdez MI (2010) Expression of IL-6, IL-8, TNF-alpha, IL-10, HSP-60, anti-HSP-60 antibodies, and anti-sperm antibodies, in semen of men with leukocytes and/or bacteria. Am J Reprod Immunol N Y N 63:233–243. doi:10.1111/j.1600-0897.2009.00786.x
58. Martorell M, Gil-Salom M, Pérez-Vallés A, Garcia JA, Rausell N, Senpere A (2005) Presence of human papillomavirus DNA in testicular biopsies from nonobstructive azoospermic men. Arch Pathol Lab Med 129:1132–1136. doi:10.1043/1543-2165(2005)129[1132:POHPDI]2.0.CO;2
59. Mazzoli S, Cai T, Addonisio P, Bechi A, Mondaini N, Bartoletti R (2010) Chlamydia trachomatis infection is related to poor semen quality in young prostatitis patients. Eur Urol 57:708–714. doi:10.1016/j.eururo.2009.05.015
60. Mazzoli S, Cai T, Rupealta V, Gavazzi A, Castricchi Pagliai R, Mondaini N, Bartoletti R (2007) Interleukin 8 and anti-chlamydia trachomatis mucosal IgA as urogenital immunologic markers in patients with C. trachomatis prostatic infection. Eur Urol 51:1385–1393. doi:10.1016/j.eururo.2006.10.059
61. McNeal JE (1988) Normal histology of the prostate. Am J Surg Pathol 12:619–633

62. Meares EM, Stamey TA (1968) Bacteriologic localization patterns in bacterial prostatitis and urethritis. Invest Urol 5:492–518

63. Mehik A, Hellström P, Lukkarinen O, Sarpola A, Järvelin M (2000) Epidemiology of prostatitis in Finnish men: a population based cross-sectional study. BJU Int 86:443–448

64. Menkveld R, Huwe P, Ludwig M, Weidner W (2003) Morphological sperm alternations in different types of prostatitis. Andrologia 35:288–293

65. Motrich RD, Maccioni M, Molina R, Tissera A, Olmedo J, Riera CM, Rivero VE (2005) Reduced semen quality in chronic prostatitis patients that have cellular autoimmune response to prostate antigens. Hum Reprod Oxf Engl 20:2567–2572. doi:10.1093/humrep/dei073

66. NHS (2014) National Health Service. NHS choices – Infertility. http://www.nhs.uk/conditions/Infertility/Pages/Introduction.aspx. Accessed 18 Jun 2015

67. Nickel JC (1998) Effective office management of chronic prostatitis. Urol Clin North Am 25:677–684

68. Nickel JC, Shoskes D, Wang Y, Alexander RB, Fowler JE, Zeitlin S, O'Leary MP, Pontari MA, Schaeffer AJ, Landis JR, Nyberg L, Kusek JW, Propert KJ (2006) How does the pre-massage and post-massage 2-glass test compare to the Meares-Stamey 4-glass test in men with chronic prostatitis/chronic pelvic pain syndrome? J Urol 176:119–124. doi:10.1016/S0022-5347(06)00498-8

69. Ochsendorf FR (1999) Infections in the male genital tract and reactive oxygen species. Hum Reprod Update 5:399–420

70. Ochsendorf FR (2008) Sexually transmitted infections: impact on male fertility. Andrologia 40:72–75. doi:10.1111/j.1439-0272.2007.00825.x

71. Onemu SO, Ibeh IN (2001) Studies on the significance of positive bacterial semen cultures in male fertility in Nigeria. Int J Fertil Womens Med 46:210–214

72. Owen DH, Katz DF (2005) A review of the physical and chemical properties of human semen and the formulation of a semen simulant. J Androl 26:459–469. doi:10.2164/jandrol.04104

73. Park H, Sim S, Lee G (2015) The presence of Chlamydia is associated with increased leukocyte counts and pain severity in men with chronic pelvic pain syndrome. Urology 85:574–579. doi:10.1016/j.urology.2014.11.008

74. Pasqualotto FF, Sharma RK, Potts JM, Nelson DR, Thomas AJ, Agarwal A (2000) Seminal oxidative stress in patients with chronic prostatitis. Urology 55:881–885

75. Perino A, Giovannelli L, Schillaci R, Ruvolo G, Fiorentino FP, Alimondi P, Cefalù E, Ammatuna P (2011) Human papillomavirus infection in couples undergoing in vitro fertilization procedures: impact on reproductive outcomes. Fertil Steril 95:1845–1848. doi:10.1016/j.fertnstert.2010.11.047

76. Practice Committee of American Society for Reproductive Medicine in collaboration with Society for Reproductive Endocrinology and Infertility (2008) Optimizing natural fertility. Fertil Steril 90:S1–S6. doi:10.1016/j.fertnstert.2008.08.122

77. Ross JDC, Jensen JS (2006) Mycoplasma genitalium as a sexually transmitted infection: implications for screening, testing, and treatment. Sex Transm Infect 82:269–271. doi:10.1136/sti.2005.017368

78. Rusz A, Pilatz A, Wagenlehner F, Linn T, Diemer T, Schuppe HC, Lohmeyer J, Hossain H, Weidner W (2012) Influence of urogenital infections and inflammation on semen quality and male fertility. World J Urol 30:23–30. doi:10.1007/s00345-011-0726-8

79. Schaeffer AJ (1999) Prostatitis: US perspective. Int J Antimicrob Agents 11:205–211; discussion 213–216

80. Schaeffer AJ, Knauss JS, Landis JR, Propert KJ, Alexander RB, Litwin MS, Nickel JC, O'Leary MP, Nadler RB, Pontari MA, Shoskes DA, Zeitlin SI, Fowler JE, Mazurick CA, Kusek JW, Nyberg LM, Chronic Prostatitis Collaborative Research Network Study Group (2002) Leukocyte and bacterial counts do not correlate with severity of symptoms in men with chronic prostatitis: the National Institutes of Health Chronic Prostatitis Cohort Study. J Urol 168:1048–1053. doi:10.1097/01.ju.0000024762.69326.df

81. Schaeffer AJ, National Institute of Diabetes and Digestive and Kidney Diseases of the US National Institutes of Health (2004) NIDDK-sponsored chronic prostatitis collaborative

research network (CPCRN) 5-year data and treatment guidelines for bacterial prostatitis. Int J Antimicrob Agents 24(Suppl 1):S49–S52. doi:10.1016/j.ijantimicag.2004.02.009

82. Schmitt M, Depuydt C, Stalpaert M, Pawlita M (2014) Bead-based multiplex sexually transmitted infection profiling. J Infect 69:123–133. doi:10.1016/j.jinf.2014.04.006

83. Schneider H, Ludwig M, Hossain HM, Diemer T, Weidner W (2003) The 2001 Giessen Cohort Study on patients with prostatitis syndrome – an evaluation of inflammatory status and search for microorganisms 10 years after a first analysis. Andrologia 35:258–262. doi:10.1046/j.1439-0272.2003.00586.x

84. Schulz M, Sánchez R, Soto L, Risopatrón J, Villegas J (2010) Effect of Escherichia coli and its soluble factors on mitochondrial membrane potential, phosphatidylserine translocation, viability, and motility of human spermatozoa. Fertil Steril 94:619–623. doi:10.1016/j.fertnstert.2009.01.140

85. Sharma RK, Pasqualotto AE, Nelson DR, Thomas AJ, Agarwal A (2001) Relationship between seminal white blood cell counts and oxidative stress in men treated at an infertility clinic. J Androl 22:575–583

86. Smelov V, Arroyo Mühr LS, Bzhalava D, Brown LJ, Komyakov B, Dillner J (2014) Metagenomic sequencing of expressed prostate secretions. J Med Virol 86:2042–2048. doi:10.1002/jmv.23900

87. Smelov V, Perekalina T, Gorelov A, Smelova N, Artemenko N, Norman L (2004) In vitro activity of fluoroquinolones, azithromycin and doxycycline against chlamydia trachomatis cultured from men with chronic lower urinary tract symptoms. Eur Urol 46:647–650. doi:10.1016/j.eururo.2004.06.020

88. Smit M, Dohle GR, Hop WCJ, Wildhagen MF, Weber RFA, Romijn JC (2007) Clinical correlates of the biological variation of sperm DNA fragmentation in infertile men attending an andrology outpatient clinic. Int J Androl 30:48–55. doi:10.1111/j.1365-2605.2006.00710.x

89. Stanford JB, Dunson DB (2007) Effects of sexual intercourse patterns in time to pregnancy studies. Am J Epidemiol 165:1088–1095. doi:10.1093/aje/kwk111

90. Taylor-Robinson D, Jensen JS (2011) Mycoplasma genitalium: from Chrysalis to multicolored butterfly. Clin Microbiol Rev 24:498–514. doi:10.1128/CMR.00006-11

91. Thonneau P, Marchand S, Tallec A, Ferial ML, Ducot B, Lansac J, Lopes P, Tabaste JM, Spira A (1991) Incidence and main causes of infertility in a resident population (1,850,000) of three French regions (1988–1989). Hum Reprod Oxf Engl 6:811–816

92. Verkooyen RP, Noordhoek GT, Klapper PE, Reid J, Schirm J, Cleator GM, Ieven M, Hoddevik G (2003) Reliability of nucleic acid amplification methods for detection of Chlamydia trachomatis in urine: results of the first international collaborative quality control study among 96 laboratories. J Clin Microbiol 41:3013–3016

93. Wagenlehner F, Pilatz A, Linn T, Diemer T, Schuppe HC, Schagdarsurengin U, Hossain H, Meinhardt A, Ellem S, Risbridger G, Weidner W (2013) Prostatitis and andrological implications. Minerva Urol E Nefrol Ital J Urol Nephrol 65:117–123

94. Weidner W, Diemer T, Wagenlehner F (2010) Male infertility in chronic urogenital infections and inflammation with special reference to ejaculate findings. In: Björndahl L, Giwercman A, Tournaye H, Weidner W (eds). Clinical andrology. EAU/ESAU course guidelines. Informa Healthcare, London, pp 293–300

95. Weidner W, Krause W, Ludwig M (1999) Relevance of male accessory gland infection for subsequent fertility with special focus on prostatitis. Hum Reprod Update 5:421–432. doi:10.1093/humupd/5.5.421

96. Weidner W, Schiefer HG, Krauss H, Jantos C, Friedrich HJ, Altmannsberger M (1991) Chronic prostatitis: a thorough search for etiologically involved microorganisms in 1,461 patients. Infection 19(Suppl 3):S119–S125

97. WHO (2000) World Health Organization. WHO manual for the standardized investigation, diagnosis and management of the infertile male. Cambridge University Press, Cambridge

98. WHO (2013) World Health Organization. Sexually transmitted infections (STIs). c2015. http://www.who.int/mediacentre/factsheets/fs110/en. Accessed 5 Jun 2015

99. World Health Organization (2010) WHO laboratory manual for the examination and processing of human semen 2010, 5th edn. WHO Press, Geneva
100. Yoon BI, Kim S, Han D-S, Ha U-S, Lee S-J, Kim HW, Han C-H, Cho Y-H (2012) Acute bacterial prostatitis: how to prevent and manage chronic infection? J Infect Chemother Off J Jpn Soc Chemother 18:444–450. doi:10.1007/s10156-011-0350-y
101. Zaneveld LJ, Tauber PF (1981) Contribution of prostatic fluid components to the ejaculate. Prog Clin Biol Res 75A:265–277
102. Zegers-Hochschild F, Adamson GD, de Mouzon J, Ishihara O, Mansour R, Nygren K, Sullivan E, van der Poel S, International Committee for Monitoring Assisted Reproductive Technology, World Health Organization (2009) The International Committee for Monitoring Assisted Reproductive Technology (ICMART) and the World Health Organization (WHO) Revised Glossary on ART Terminology, 2009. Hum Reprod Oxf Engl 24:2683–2687. doi:10.1093/humrep/dep343
103. Zermann DH, Ishigooka M, Doggweiler R, Schmidt RA (1999) Neurourological insights into the etiology of genitourinary pain in men. J Urol 161:903–908
104. Zohdy W (2009) Clinical parameters that predict successful outcome in men with premature ejaculation and inflammatory prostatitis. J Sex Med 6:3139–3146. doi:10.1111/j.1743-6109. 2009.01487.x

Elevated PSA as Differential Diagnostic Error-Source in Prostate Cancer with Consequences in Medical Law

14

Karl-Horst Bichler and Kurt G. Naber

14.1 Introduction

Misinterpretation of elevated serum prostatic-specific antigen (PSA) levels due to urinary tract infection (UTI) or prostatitis can lead to serious complications in patients with prostate cancer. In addition to digital rectal examination (DRE) of the prostate gland and transrectal sonography (TRUS), measurement of the antigen plays an important role in the diagnosis of prostate cancer.

Wrong steps are, for example:

(i) Elevated PSA level (>10 ng/ml) without suspicious palpation incorrectly associated with UTI or prostatitis and subsequent antibiotic therapy
(ii) Assumed but not correctly diagnosed prostatitis with elevated PSA and repeated negative prostate biopsies

Two case studies from our experience in medical law demonstrate these problems.

K.-H. Bichler
Professor em. of Urology, University of Tuebingen,
Oskar Schlemmerstr. 5, 70191, Stuttgart, Germany
e-mail: khbichler@web.de

K.G. Naber (✉)
Professor of Urology, Technical University of Munich,
Karl-Bickleder-Str. 44, 94315, Stuttgart, Germany
e-mail: kurt@nabers.de

© Springer International Publishing Switzerland 2016
T. Cai, T.E. Bjerklund Johansen (eds.), *Prostatitis and Its Management: Concepts and Recommendations for Clinical Practice*, DOI 10.1007/978-3-319-25175-2_14

14.2 Case 1

A 53-year-old man presented with bladder-emptying disorder and "urine stream weakening" associated with a slightly enlarged prostate due to benign prostatic hyperplasia (BPH). The examination revealed "UTI" with "many" leukocytes in the urine, bacteriuria due to *Enterobacter cloacae*, and an elevated serum PSA level of 20 ng/ml. DRE did not show any induration suspect of cancer. The urologist explained the elevated PSA level with UTI or prostatitis and initiated antibiotic treatment (piperacillin/tazobactam). Clinical symptoms indicative of UTI or prostatitis were not mentioned in the medical record. In addition, the urologist prescribed medication to improve bladder voiding (tamsulosin) and treatment of BPH with a 5-alpha reductase inhibitor (finasteride).

Control visits after 4 and 12 weeks revealed again "suspicion of UTI with many leucocytes." Treatment was continued with antibiotics and with medication for bladder voiding and reduction of BPH. After 4 months, the PSA level showed only a small decrease to 17.8 ng/ml. Three weeks later, the urologist recorded his telephone call to the patient as follows: "Prostate biopsy necessary! The patient is unreasonable and does not agree."

Two and a half months later, the patient visited the urologist again. He did not want a physical examination but only a new prescription of his previous medication. In the record, it was not mentioned that on this occasion the patient was made aware by several means of the suspected prostate cancer diagnosis, nor was the patient's family physician informed accordingly.

Four years later, the patient's physician referred him again to the urologist because of a high PSA level, now measuring 300 ng/ml! The DRE revealed a hard prostate, very suspicious of cancer also considering the high PSA level. The subsequent biopsy discovered a carcinoma of the prostate (Gleason 9). Radical surgery showed an advanced prostate tumor (pT3b) with tumorous tissue in both lobes of the prostate, infiltration of the seminal vesicles, and regional lymph node metastases.

In summary, the patient was urologically examined because of his voiding problems due to BPH. A clearly elevated PSA level, leukocyturia, and bacteriuria (without reported symptoms) were found. The DRE of the prostate was not suspicious of cancer. Wrongly, the urologist associated the PSA elevation with UTI and initiated antibiotic treatment (piperacillin/tazobactam) and medical therapy of the voiding disturbances. There was, however, no significant reduction of the PSA in the following several months and still no biopsies were performed for histological clarification. Thereafter, the patient withdrew from urological follow-up. Four years later, he returned with a PSA level of 300 ng//ml and a biopsy revealed carcinoma of the prostate. The question arises: Is antibiotic therapy justified in cases of elevated PSA (>10 ng/ml) when UTI or prostatitis is suspected but not confirmed with adequate diagnostic measures?

14.3 Case 2

A 59-year-old man with a 3-year history of elevated PSA levels of around 30 ng/ml was found to have a prostate of firm consistency on DRE. Exprimate urine contained many leucocytes. Because of highly suspected cancer, three sets of prostate biopsies were performed over the years, each time without any evidence of a tumor. Therefore, the urologist assumed that the elevated PSA was due to "prostatitis." But no relevant clinical symptoms of either acute or chronic prostatitis had been recorded and no further specific diagnostic procedures in this direction were carried out. The patient received repeated courses of antibiotic treatment.

When hematuria occurred, a cystoscopy and a transrectal ultrasonography were performed. By sonography, an enlarged prostate with an adjoining tumor area was found. Endoscopic examination revealed a stilted exophytic tumor of the colliculus seminalis growing toward the bladder. The tumor was resected transurethrally. Histologic examination showed a prostate cancer originating from the prostatic urethra or colliculus seminalis growing toward the bladder, a so-called ductal carcinoma of the prostate gland.

In summary, during 3 years, highly significant PSA elevations were observed. Because of suspicious DRE, a prostate cancer was suspected, and in the course of time, repeated prostate biopsies were carried out, none of which indicated tumors. Because of pyuria in the exprimate urine, prostatitis was assumed and the patient was treated with antibiotics [2].

14.4 PSA Elevation in Prostatitis/Epididymitis and Urinary Tract Infection

Regarding the connection between UTI/prostatitis/epididymitis and PSA elevation, the question of pathogenesis must be raised. PSA is a specific marker (protease) of the prostate tissue. The antigen is produced by the epithelial cells of the prostate gland and drained into the ductuli. Here, the protease plays a role in the liquidification of seminal coagula [31]. A stimulating androgen effect on PSA formation exists (gene activation). The usual normal serum level of PSA is <4 ng/ml. However, the upper limit is also age specific: <50 years 2.5 ng/ml; 50–59 years 3.5 ng/ml; 60–69 years 4.5 ng/ml; 70–79 years 6.5 ng/ml [32].

Different kinds of damage of the prostate cells, e.g., infection, inflammation, malignant degeneration, or other injuries, lead to the release of PSA into the stroma of the organ. From there, it enters the vascular system via lymphatic vessels. Elevated serum PSA levels appear in prostatitis, BPH (increased volume), and especially in prostate cancer. Febrile UTI, even without characteristic prostatic pain, can raise PSA levels, although in such cases, an inflamed prostate is expected [40]. How high PSA elevation that can be anticipated in asymptomatic bacteriuria, for example, in patients with indwelling catheter or in lower UTI, has not yet been documented in convincing studies.

An acute or chronic inflammatory process of the prostate gland can cause a pathologic elevation of the PSA level without clinical signs and symptoms of prostatitis [13, 16, 27]. This is explained by the release of PSA from the prostatic cells damaged by inflammation. If a PSA level is above normal age range and an inflammatory prostate process is assumed, relevant examinations are necessary to establish the diagnosis of an acute or chronic bacterial prostatitis before any antibiotic therapy is initiated.

Patients with acute bacterial prostatitis complain of typical clinical symptoms of acute UTI with irritative and/or obstructive voiding disturbances. Frequently, they also have symptoms of a systemic infection with fatigue, nausea, vomiting, fever, chills, and even urosepsis. In addition, there can be perineal and suprapubic pain which can radiate to the outer genitals. On digital-rectal examination, patients complain of strong tenderness of the prostate. Massage of the prostate is contraindicated since this can cause sepsis [1, 10]. The bacteriological examination is done with mid-stream urine. Infravesical obstructions or an intraprostatic abscess have to be ruled out or treated accordingly. Following diagnosis, an immediate broad spectrum antibiotic therapy including all measures required is necessary [12, 28].

The diagnostics of chronic-bacterial prostatitis should include medical history, registration of symptoms according to the NIH symptom score, a standardized microscopic and bacteriological analysis using the four glass test (first-voided urine, midstream urine, prostate secretion after prostate massage and prostate exprimate urine), or a two-glass test (midstream urine and exprimate urine) [20, 23, 25, 30]. Suspicious findings (e.g., erythrocyturia) require urethrocystoscopy and/or transrectal ultrasonography [2].

Elevated PSA levels due to UTI raise the question whether this antigen, a protease, originates also from other organs than the prostate, especially from renal and urinary tract structures. Evidence of PSA in extraprostatic tissue was provided by immune reaction in the urethra, in the periurethral glands (male and female), and in adenoid cell carcinomas of the urethra and urinary bladder [3]. Schmidt et al. [35] detected PSA (mean 0.29 ng/ml) in the urine of 11 % of 217 women without sexual intercourse during the last 48 h. The detection of PSA in the urethra and urinary bladder, however, is fairly weak and not constant. This phenomenon is due to different specificity and sensitivity of the antibodies used [3].

Concerning the pathogenesis of elevated PSA levels due to inflammatory changes of the urinary tract, the studies of Ulleryd et al. [38] are important. In 83 % of 70 male patients with febrile UTI, the authors found elevated PSA levels with a median of 14 ng/ml (range 0.54–140 ng/ml). The patients had at least one of the typical symptoms of an acute UTI, such as dysuria, flank pain, fever of at least 38 °C and a significant bacteriuria, mainly due to E. coli [17]. Only six (9 %) of the patients complained of pain during DRE of the prostate. These investigations show that the prostate in men is involved during febrile UTI episodes which are demonstrated by elevated PSA levels [40]. In contrast, serum PSA levels were not above 1 ng/ml in 16 control patients with febrile infections of other origin.

Pilatz et al. [33] investigated 237 patients with acute epididymitis concerning etiology and outcome. PSA levels dropped within 3 months from a mean of 2.1 (range 0.8–5.6) ng/ml in antibiotic-naive patients to about half of the initial values in those cases with detected bacterial pathogens but remained more or less stable in those cases without evidence for bacterial pathogens. In pretreated patients, PSA levels declined to a similar extent, as witnessed in antibiotic-naive patients with pathogens, irrespective of whether a pathogen was detected or not. In patients where pathogen detection was based on 16S rDNA analysis, PSA values declined to a comparable degree. Elevated PSA levels in epididymitis may be explained by the fact that epididymitis is usually considered an ascending infection from the prostate.

> Thus, it can be stated that significant elevated PSA levels are always caused by alterations of the prostatic cells, the origin of the antigen. The extraprostatic origin of PSA, especially from renal and urinary tract structures, is uncertain. An elevated PSA always stands for a causal involvement of the prostate.

In febrile UTI (i.e., body temperature of 38 °C or more, flank pain, with or without painful palpation of the prostate, and significant bacteriuria with cfu $\geq 10^4$/ml due to *E. coli*), the prostate (prostatitis) is often involved as documented by distinct elevated PSA levels. In asymptomatic bacteriuria with or without leukocyturia or in a simple lower UTI, prostatic involvement is not expected. Convincing studies, however, are missing.

14.5   Antibiotic Therapy and Increased PSA Values

PSA levels may increase due to acute or chronic bacterial prostatitis/epididymitis and/or febrile UTI and decrease again during and after antibiotic therapy, which, however, takes some time. One month after therapy, 43 % of 70 men treated for febrile UTI still showed increased PSA levels, which finally dropped to a median of 1.5. ng/ml only after 12 months. The reductions in PSA and prostate volume were significantly correlated. The slow decline of PSA levels in some patients indicates a protracted healing process, according to the authors. Interestingly, in one patient with disseminated prostate cancer who had raised baseline levels of PSA responded to the infection with a further increase in serum PSA, which was interpreted in a way that different prostatic affections may have an additive effect on PSA levels [38, 39].

On this background, it was assumed that the part of PSA, which is increased due to infection, can be reduced to normal after the infection is cured by a suitable antibiotic therapy, whereas the part of PSA increased due to a concomitant prostatic cancer will remain the same. Later on, however, antibiotic therapy was not only performed, in case of bacterial prostatitis (acute or chronic) or febrile UTI, but also for any kind of elevated PSA as sort of differential therapy to reduce that part of PSA, which was probably increased due to infectious microfoci. If the PSA levels returned to normal after therapy, no prostatic biopsy was needed. This approach seemed to be even more justified, because increased PSA levels have also been found in asymptomatic inflammatory changes of the prostate [13, 19]. Serretta et al. [36] treated 99 patients due to elevated PSA for 3 weeks with ciprofloxacin. In 65 % of cases, histology detected small foci of prostatitis. No cancer was detected if PSA decreased below 4 ng/ml or more than 70 %. Nickel et al. [29], however, could not find any correlation between kind and grade of inflammation and the total PSA or PSA density in patients with BPH and LUTS. The PSA increase in BPH patients was mainly explained by hyperplasia and not so much by the asymptomatic prostatitis [16, 24, 26].

It could be shown in several studies that a statistically significant PSA reduction could also be achieved by antibiotic therapy in asymptomatic patients with or without inflammatory changes, e.g., increased leukocytes in prostatic secretion or histological inflammation [4, 6, 7, 11, 16, 21, 34]. According to these authors, this could make prostate biopsies unnecessary. Although most of the authors requested to establish such recommendations by further studies, this approach was widely and uncritically used in clinical practice [41].

Other investigators have interpreted their results more carefully. Although they could also demonstrate reduction of PSA levels after antibiotic therapy, they concluded that the accuracy of this finding was not sufficient to save prostatic biopsies if indicated [8, 9, 14, 37] or such findings could only be interpreted in connection with other features [22]. Finally, Kim et al. [15] demonstrated in their study including 86 men with initial PSA values between 4.6 and 24.8 ng/ml and with increased leukocytes in prostatic secretion that with a 4-week antibiotic therapy, the PSA values could be decreased by about one third, but that in 5/37 (13.5 %) of the patients with a PSA <4 ng/ml as compared to13/49 (26.5 %) with a PSA >4 ng/ml a prostate cancer could still be detected later by biopsy.

Bruyère and Lakmichi [5] performed an extended literature review of the last 20 years and concluded that a systematic antibiotic use to reduce increased PSA levels to save prostatic biopsies must be considered irrelevant and will propagate only antibiotic resistance. Whether more sophisticated PSA diagnostics could probably improve differentiation between prostate cancer on one side and BPH and inflammation/infection on the other remains to be investigated [18].

14.6   Evaluation of the Case Reports

Case 1 is a good example showing that any PSA increase of more than 10 ng/ml above the age range is highly suspicious of prostate cancer even in a patient with concomitant signs and probably symptoms (not mentioned) of lower, nonfebrile UTI. To explain such a PSA increase only by laboratory findings, such as leukocyturia and bacteriuria, as in this case is absolutely careless. If a bacterial prostatitis (acute or chronic) is considered a differential diagnosis, appropriate investigations, e.g., four-glass test, have to be performed to establish or exclude such a diagnosis.

Therefore, the first mistake in this case was to assume that laboratory findings, such as leukocyturia and bacteriuria, and probably symptoms of lower UTI (not mentioned) explain the increased PSA levels sufficiently and justify therefore long-term antibiotic therapy, although neither acute nor chronic bacterial prostatitis was positively diagnosed. Consequently, the final diagnosis of prostate cancer was postponed far too long.

The second mistake was that the patient was not informed about the urologist's differential diagnosis, regardless that this differential diagnosis later proved to be wrong. However, if the patient had been informed as early as possible about the highly possible existence of a prostate cancer and thus a much more severe disease, he had most likely insisted on a sooner final diagnosis.

Finally, the third mistake was that the urologist did not inform the family physician or the patient about his differential diagnosis and treatment approach. There would have been a chance of an alert general physician to recommend the patient to go for a second opinion.

All these mistakes caused that a final diagnosis was made too late. The urologist's later telephone call for a second visit could not possibly be understood by the patient as a possible more serious diagnosis such as a prostate cancer. The urologist should have included the patient in his differential diagnosis of a prostate cancer right from the beginning, and the family physician should have been informed about this.

In case 2 taken from Bichler and Wechsel [2], because of severely pathologically elevated PSA levels, the urologists performed several prostate biopsies in accordance with the current guidelines. These failed, however, to demonstrate prostate cancer. Therefore, the urologists assumed a prostatitis causing the elevated PSA. Unfortunately, they did not perform the investigations requested according to the guidelines to diagnose a prostatitis, e.g., four-glass test in case of chronic bacterial prostatitis [10]. In such a complex situation with striking laboratory findings in the urine (erythrocyturia) and in the exprimate, the urologist should have performed further investigations, such as urethrocystoscopy and transrectal ultrasonography. The final diagnosis of a ductal carcinoma of the prostate was not reached until a urethrocystoscopy was performed due to hematuria.

Although the urologists followed primarily the guidelines concerning the prostate biopsies, their misinterpretation of elevated PSA as caused by prostatitis in case of negative biopsies led to the yearlong protraction of the final diagnosis of a prostate cancer. Prostatitis, however, was only assumed but not diagnosed according to the established guidelines. The difficult morphological characteristics may be acknowledged in this case, which hampered the diagnosis of a ductal carcinoma by transrectal biopsy.

This case also demonstrates that under strong suspicion of prostate cancer, it is not enough to follow the guidelines with DRE and prostate biopsies. To clarify considerably elevated PSA levels, further investigations are sometimes needed. The alibi diagnosis of prostatitis without appropriate clarification was insufficient. Therefore, a treatment failure by the finally responsible urologist had to be supposed, because the assumed prostatitis as cause for the elevated PSA was not properly diagnosed.

Conclusions

These two case reports demonstrate possible errors that can be made when elevated PSA levels are thought to stem from urogenital infections which are diagnosed based on pathological laboratory findings only, e.g., leukocyturia and bacteriuria, although a positively diagnosed prostatitis (acute or chronic) or a febrile UTI could not be demonstrated. Consequently in the first case, the inevitable prostate biopsy was protracted by a useless antibiotic therapy far too long. In the second case, negative prostate biopsies misled to the same wrong concept that antibiotic therapy might be indicated "to treat" elevated PSA levels without a proven diagnosis of an acute or chronic bacterial prostatitis or febrile UTI. Other forms of prostate cancer and additional diagnostic measures were ignored. In both cases, the final diagnosis of prostate cancer was unjustifiably protracted for too long.

In the spirit of a positive error management culture, it is important to search for sources of errors and carefully discuss typical mistakes and possible underlying misconceptions. It should be discussed why such mistakes could happen and how such mistakes can be avoided in the future [2].

Take-Home Message
- Elevated PSA levels without alteration of the prostate are not allegeable.
- Considerably elevated PSA levels are always suspicious for prostate cancer.
- Febrile UTIs (body temperature ≥ 38 °C with corresponding symptoms) often show involvement of the prostate as demonstrated by elevated PSA levels.
- Asymptomatic bacteriuria or simple lower UTI is not accountable for elevated PSA.
- If a prostatitis (acute or chronic) is assumed as causative for elevated PSA levels, an appropriate diagnostic clarification is necessary, e.g., four-glass test.
- Ex juvantibus antibiotic differential therapy to possibly "lower elevated PSA to normal" and thus saving prostate biopsy is not indicated any more.
- Insistent information of the patient and documentation are essential from the beginning to avoid protraction of the diagnosis and patient's drifting off.

References

1. Bichler K-H (2004) Das Urologische Gutachten, 2nd edn. Springer, Berlin
2. Bichler K-H, Wechsel HW (2011) Urologische Begutachtung im Arzthaftpflichtverfahren. Sammlung typischer Kasuistiken. Lehmanns Media, Berlin. ISBN 978-3-86541-424-3
3. Bostwick DG (1977) Urologic surgical pathology. Mosby/St. Louis, Missouri
4. Bozeman CB, Carves BS, Eastam JA, Venable DD (2002) Treatment of chronic prostatitis lowers serum prostate specific antigen. J Urol 167:1723–1726
5. Bruyère F, Lakmichi AM (2013) PSA interest and prostatitis: literature review. (Article in French). Prog Urol 23:1377–1381

6. Del Rosso A, Saldutto P, Di Pierro ED, Masciovecchio S, Galatioto GP, Vicentini C (2012) Impacts of antibiotic and anti-inflammatory therapy on serum prostate specific antigen in asymptomatic men: our experience. (Article in Italian). Urologia 79(Suppl 19):37–40

7. Dirim A, Tekin ML, Koyluoglu E, Oguzulgen AI, Peskircioglu L, Ozkardes H (2009) Do changes in a high serum prostate-specific antigen level and the free/total prostate-specific anti-gen ratio after antibiotic treatment rule out biopsy and the suspicion of cancer? Urol Int 82:266–269

8. Eggener SE, Large MC, Gerber GS, Pettus J, Yossepowitch O, Smith ND, Kundu S, Kunnavakkam R, Zorn K, Raman JD (2013) Empiric antibiotics for an elevated prostate-specific antigen (PSA) level: a randomised, prospective, controlled multi-institutional trial. BJU Int 112(7):925–929

9. Faydaci G, Eryildirim B, Tarhan F, Goktas C, Tosun C, Kuyumcuoglu U (2012) Does antibio-therapy prevent unnecessary prostate biopsies in patients with high PSA values? [Article in Spanish]. Actas Urol Esp 36(4):234–238

10. Grabe M, Bjerklund-Johansen TE, Bartoletti R, Çek M, Naber KG, Pickard RS, Tenke P, Wagenlehner F, Wullt B. Guidelines on urological infections. Part 19, pp 1–107. European Association of Urology 2014, Arnhem, ISBN 978-90-79754-65-6. http://www.uroweb.org/gls/pdf/19%20Urological%20infections_LR.pdf

11. Guercio S, Terrone C, Tarabuzzi R, Poggio M, Cracco C, Bollito E, Scarpa RM (2004) PSA decrease after levofloxacin therapy in patients with histological prostatitis. Arch Ital Urol Androl 76(4):154–158

12. Ha U-S und Y-H Cho. Acute bacterial prostatitis. In: Naber KG, Schaeffer AJ, Heyns CH, Matsumoto T, Shoskes DA, Bjerklund Johanses TE (eds). Urogenital infections. European Association of Urology – International Consultation on Urological Diseases, Edition 2010, pp 714–727. Arnhem, ISBN: 978-90-79754-41-0 http://www.icud.info/urogenitalinfections.html. Visited 19 July 2014

13. Hasui Y, Marutsuka K, Asada Y, Ide H, Nishi S, Osada Y (1994) Relationship between serum prostate specific antigen and histological prostatitis in patients with benign prostatic hyperpla-sia. Prostate 25(2):91–96

14. Hochreiter WW (2008) The issue of prostate cancer evaluation in men with elevated prostate-specific antigen and chronic prostatitis. Andrologia 40(2):130–133

15. Kim YJ, Kim SO, Ryu KH, Hwang IS, Hwang EC, Oh KJ, Jung SI, Kang TW, Kwon DD, Park K, Ryu SB (2011) Prostate cancer can be detected even in patients with decreased PSA less than 2.5 ng/ml after treatment of chronic prostatitis. Korean J Urol 52(7):457–460

16. Kyung Y-S, Lee H-C, Kim H-J (2010) Changes in serum prostate-specific antigen after treat-ment with antibiotics in patients with lower urinary tract symptoms/benign prostatic hyperpla-sia with prostatitis. Int Neurourol J 14:100–104

17. Johnson JR, Scheutz F, Ulleryd P, Kuskowski MA, O'Bryan TT, Sandberg T (2005) Host-pathogen relationships among Escherichia coli isolates recovered from men with febrile uri-nary tract infection. Clin Inf Dis 40:813–822

18. Lazzeri M, Abrate A, Lughezzani G, Gadda GM, Freschi M, Mistretta F, Lista G, Fossati N, Larcher A, Kinzikeeva E, Buffi N, Dell'Acqua V, Bini V, Montorsi F, Guazzoni G (2014) Relationship of chronic histologic prostatic inflammation in biopsy specimens with serum iso-form [−2]proPSA (p2PSA), %p2PSA, and prostate health index in men with a total prostate-specific antigen of 4–10 ng/ml and normal digital rectal examination. Urology 83(3):606–612

19. Liotta RF, Tarantino ML, Melloni D (2008) Chronic prostatitis and PSA values. [Article in Italian]. Urologia 75(1):102–104

20. Litwin MS, McNaughton-Collins M, Fowler FJ Jr, Nickel JC, Calhoun E, Pontari MA, Alexander RB, Farrar JT, O'Leary MP, The Chronic Prostatitis Collaborative Research Network (1999) The National Institutes of Health chronic prostatitis symptom index. J Urol 162:369–475

21. Lorente JA, Arango O, Bielsa O, Cortadellas R, Gelabert-Mas A (2002) Effect of antibi-otic treatment on serum PSA and percent free PSA levels in patients with biochemical criteria for prostate biopsy and previous lower urinary tract infections. Int J Biol Markers 17(2):84–9

22. Magri V, Trinchieri A, Montanari E, Del Nero A, Mangiarotti B, Zirpoli P, de Eguileor M, Marras E, Ceriani I, Vral A, Perletti G (2007) Reduction of PSA values by combination pharmacological therapy in patients with chronic prostatitis: implications for prostate cancer detection. Arch Ital Urol Androl 79(2):84–92
23. Meares EM, Stamey TA (1968) Bacteriologic localization patterns in bacterial prostatitis and urethritis. Invest Urol 5(5):492–518
24. Morote J, Lopez M, Encabo G, de Torres IM (2000) Effect of inflammation and benign prostatic enlargement on total and percent free serum prostatic specific antigen. Eur Urol 37(5):537–540
25. Wagenlehner FME, Naber KG, Weidner W (2008) Prostatitis, epididymitis, and orchitis. In: Cohen J, Powderly WG, Opal SM (eds) Infectious Diseases. 3rd edition, chapter 54, Saunders, Elsevier, 2008
26. Nadler RB, Humphrey PA, Smith DS, Catalona WJ, Ratliff TL (1995) Effect of inflammation and benign prostatic hyperplasia on elevated serum prostate specific antigen levels. J Urol 154(2 Pt 1):407–413
27. Neal DE Jr, Clejan S, Sarma D, Moon TD (1992) Prostate specific antigen and prostatitis. I. Effect of prostatitis on serum PSA in the human and nonhuman primate. Prostate 20(2):105–111
28. Neal DE Jr (1999) Treatment of acute prostatitis. In: Nickel JC (ed) Textbook of prostatitis. Isis Medical Media, Oxford
29. Nickel JC, Downey J, Young I, Boag S (1999) Asymptomatic inflammation and/or infection in benign prostatic hyperplasia. BJU Int 84(9):976–981
30. Nickel JC, Shoskes D, Wang Y, Alexander RB, Fowler JE Jr, Zeitlin S, O'Leary MP, Pontari MA, Schaeffer AJ, Landis JR, Nyberg L, Kusek JW, Propert KJ, Chronic Prostatitis Collaborative Research Network Study Group (2006) How does the pre-massage and post-massage 2-glass test compare to the Meares-Stamey 4-glass test in men with chronic prostatitis/chronic pelvic pain syndrome? J Urol 176:119–124
31. Nieschlag E, Behre HM, Nieschlag S (eds) (2009) Andrology. Basics and clinic of reproductive health in man (German textbook), 3rd edn. Springer, Berlin. ISBN 978-3-540-92962-8
32. Oesterling JE (1996) Age-specific reference ranges for serum PSA. N Engl J Med 335(5):345–346
33. Pilatz A, Hossain H, Kaiser R, Mankertz A, Schuettler CG, Domann E, Schuppe H-C, Chakraborty T, Weidner W, Wagenlehner F (2014) Acute epididymitis revisited: impact of molecular diagnostics on etiology and contemporary guideline recommendations. Eur Urol. pii: S0302-2838(14)01260-3. doi:10.1016/j.eururo.2014.12.005
34. Schaeffer AJ, Wu SC, Tennenberg AM, Kahn JB (2005) Treatment of chronic bacterial prostatitis with levofloxacin and ciprofloxacin lowers serum prostate specific antigen. J Urol 174(1):161–4
35. Schmidt S, Franke M, Lehmann J, Loch T, Stöckle M, Weichert-Jacobsen K (2001) Prostate-specific antigen in female urine: a prospective study involving 217 women. Urology 57(4):717–720
36. Serretta V, Catanese A, Daricello G, Liotta R, Allegro R, Martorana A, Aragona F, Melloni D (2008) PSA reduction (after antibiotics) permits to avoid or postpone prostate biopsy in selected patients. Prostate Cancer Prostatic Dis 11(2):148–152
37. Toktas G, Demiray M, Erkan E, Kocaaslan R, Yucetas U, Unluer SE (2013) The effect of antibiotherapy on prostate-specific antigen levels and prostate biopsy results in patients with levels 2.5 to 10 ng/mL. J Endourol 27(8):1061–1067
38. Ulleryd P, Zackrisson B, Aus G, Bergdahl S, Hugosson J, Sandberg T (1999) Prostatic involvement in men with febrile urinary tract infection as measured by serum prostate-specific antigen and transrectal ultrasonography. BJU Int 84(4):470–474
39. Ulleryd P (2003) Febrile urinary tract infection in men. Int J Antimicrob Agents 22:89–93
40. Zackrisson B, Ulleryd P et al (2003) Evolution of free complexed, and total serum prostate-specific antigen and their ratios during 1 year of follow-up of men with febrile urinary tract infection. Urology 62:278–181
41. Yoo DS, Woo SH, Cho S, Kang SH, Kim SJ, Park SY, Lee SH, Jeon SH, Park J (2014) Practice patterns of urologists in managing Korean men aged 40 years or younger with high serum prostate-specific antigen levels. Urology 83(6):1339–1343

The Prostatitis Patient: "A Clinical Dialogue"

15

Tommaso Cai and Truls E. Bjerklund Johansen

In this section we would like to give the readers a practical approach to the management of the prostatitis patient. The scene is a urologist who is discussing a prostatitis patient with a colleague, a general practitioner.

Legend:
GP: *General practitioner*
UR: *Urologist*

GP. What is the prevalence of prostatitis in the outpatient setting?
UR. The prevalence of patients with prostatitis-like symptoms is reported to be about 8–13 % of all visits in an outpatient setting. Recent evidence showed an increasing prevalence of prostatitis patients during the last years. This is probably due to improved diagnostic facilities and to a better understanding of the presentation forms of the prostatitis syndrome. However, there are still aspects of the diagnostic workup that need to be improved, in particular the microbiological evaluation. In this sense, the prevalence of prostatitis patients should be considered a "tip of the iceberg" only. The recent study of the epidemiological characteristics of the disease is a very important step in the understanding of the natural history of this disease. Moreover, the analysis of epidemiological characteristics may help us improve our management of the complications of this clinical condition.

T. Cai
Department of Urology, Santa Chiara Regional Hospital, Trento, Italy
e-mail: ktommy@libero.it

T.E.B. Johansen (✉)
Department of Urology, Oslo University Hospital, Oslo, Norway

Institute of Clinical Medicine, University of Aarhus, Aarhus, Denmark
e-mail: tebj@medisin.uio.no

© Springer International Publishing Switzerland 2016
T. Cai, T.E. Bjerklund Johansen (eds.), *Prostatitis and Its Management: Concepts and Recommendations for Clinical Practice*, DOI 10.1007/978-3-319-25175-2_15

GP. You talk about the complications of prostatitis. What kind of complications can that be?

UR. The patient suffering from prostatitis can develop numerous complications related to sexual function and fertility. In more detail, a patient with bacterial prostatitis due to *Chlamydia trachomatis* infection (that is a sexually transmitted pathogen) can develop a reduction of semen quality, unless he is properly treated and cured. Other sexually transmitted pathogens, such as HPV and mycoplasmas, may also impair fertility. Therefore a thorough microbiological investigation is strongly recommended. On the other hand, some patients affected by prostatitis present with sexual symptoms like premature ejaculation and erectile dysfunction. Hence, the management of the prostatitis patient is very important in order to avoid future complications.

GP. What kind of microbiological investigation do I need to perform in a patient suspected of having prostatitis?

UR. The Meares and Stamey test is the gold standard for sampling of specimens for a microbiological evaluation of a patient with prostatitis. This is a simple test to perform, but it is able to give us crucial information about the disease. Although the Meares and Stamey 4-glass test is the standard method for assessing inflammation and the presence of bacteria in the lower urinary tract in men presenting with the chronic prostatitis syndrome, the test is rarely used, even by urologists. However, many times, we can use a simpler test, the 2-glass pre-massage and post-massage test which is more rapid to perform. The Meares and Stamey test means collection of 4 sequential urine samples. Two are taken before prostatic massage, the first from the initial 10 mL and the second from the midstream urine. After prostatic massage, drops of expressed prostatic secretion are collected, as is the first 10 mL of urine passed after massage. When bacteria, inflammatory cells, or both are significantly higher in the two samples after prostatic massage, the findings are considered pathognomonic for prostatitis. By using this test we can assign the patient to a specific category of prostatitis. Moreover, this test is also suitable to study if inflammatory cells are present in the urine and thus give us more useful data for the management of the patient.

GP. You talk about a specific category of prostatitis. Is there a classification of prostatitis that I can use in the management of my patients?

UR. Yes, there is a classification of the prostatitis syndrome which is mainly based on clinical and laboratory findings, but sometimes imaging or even histological examination is used. The recent National Institutes of Health (NIH) classification of the prostatitis syndrome includes four main categories: (1) acute bacterial prostatitis; (2) chronic bacterial prostatitis; (3) chronic prostatitis/chronic pelvic pain syndrome, (3a) inflammatory and (3b) noninflammatory; and (4) asymptomatic inflammatory prostatitis. The assessment to each category is based on the results of the Meares and Stamey test. About 10 % of prostatitis patients will have a bacterial prostatitis (category I or II), while the majority of patients demonstrate clinical and laboratory characteristics indicative of cat. III. Clearly, in category I and II antibiotic treatment is necessary, while in category III the management is very difficult and complex.

GP. What is the role of imaging in the management of the prostatitis patients?
UR. The role of imaging in the management of prostatitis patients is limited. However, in acute bacterial prostatitis patients who deteriorate and develop sepsis within 72 h, radiological investigations are mandatory to investigate possible complications. Otherwise imaging is only indicated in cases where there is suspicion of pyelonephritis and in cases with persistent local symptoms where a prostatic abscess is suspected. On the other hand, in chronic prostatitis, sonography findings may be normal or reveal nonspecific abnormalities such as: numerous calcifications in the posterolateral regions of the peripheral prostate and a non-homogenous echostructure of the prostatic parenchyma, alternating between scattered hyperechoic strips and hypoechoic zones that sometimes contain pseudonodules and dilated ducts. Increased vascularization is not detectable with standard black and white sonography equipment. The use of other imaging modalities, such as MRI, is indicated in special situations only, like when a granulomatous prostatitis is suspected. MRI is also helpful in the diagnosis of a prostatic abscess.

GP. You talk about the role of prostate calcifications. What is the importance of prostate calcifications for the management of these patients?
UR. The role of prostate calcifications is currently under debate. Several authors state that calcifications can be a marker of chronic prostate inflammation and even of acute bacterial infection. In particular, some authors argue that prostate calcifications consist of bacteria-like organisms similar to species isolated from biological materials and calcifications in other parts of the body. Moreover, authors state that bacterial strains that are able to produce biofilms are consistently present in patients with chronic bacterial prostatitis. Other authors consider the prostate calcifications a sign of previous inflammatory events and try to correlate the presence of calcifications with the patient's symptoms and the risk of disease progression. The role of prostate calcifications is very interesting, and future studies should be planned in order to further clarify this enigma.

GP. What is the correct antibiotic treatment schedule to use in patients with acute bacterial prostatitis?
UR. As the European Association of Urology (EAU) guidelines on urological infections recommend, the first-line class of antibiotics to use is: fluoroquinolones. They have a good pharmacological profile that allows a good penetration into the prostatic tissue and have a useful spectrum of activity against the most commonly isolated bacteria in these patients. In fact, the main obstacle for a successful eradication of causative pathogens is the suboptimal pharmacokinetic properties of the therapeutic agents used which prevent the efficient delivery of the drugs to

the sites of bacterial infection inside the prostate. However, you should always try to obtain results of the antibiograms from the Meares and Stamey test before an antibiotic is prescribed. As stated in the EAU guidelines, in acute bacterial prostatitis the parenteral administration of high doses of bactericidal antibiotics, such as broad-spectrum penicillin, a third-generation cephalosporin, or a fluoro-quinolone, should be given on an empirical basis. This means that antibiotics are given before the results of cultures are available. For initial therapy, any of these antibiotics may be combined with an aminoglycoside. After defervescence and normalization of infection parameters, intravenous treatment can be substituted with oral drugs and continued for a total of 2–4 weeks. The recommended anti-biotics in chronic bacterial prostatitis are again fluoroquinolones, such as cipro-floxacin and levofloxacin. They have a generally good safety profile and demonstrate antibacterial activity against Gram-negative pathogens, including *P. aeruginosa*. In addition, levofloxacin is active against Gram-positive and atypi-cal pathogens, such as *C. trachomatis* and genital mycoplasmas. The recom-mended duration of antibiotic treatment in chronic bacterial prostatitis is 4–6 weeks after initial diagnosis. Relatively high doses are needed and oral adminis-tration is preferred. If intracellular bacteria have been detected or are suspected, tetracyclines or erythromycin should be given.

GP. Can I use antibiotics in the management of nonbacterial prostatitis patients?

UR. Yes, the urologists often use antibiotics in the nonbacterial prostatitis patients, too. However, for the sake of antibiotic stewardship, the use of antibiotics should be limited to patients with confirmed bacterial prostatitis only. The rationale for the use of antibiotics in nonbacterial prostatitis is a strong clinical suspicion of a bacterial infection despite the lack of positive microbiological results. In fact, there are many cases where we are unable to identify specific bacterial strains. Whenever antibiotics are prescribed in nonbacterial prostatitis, the effect should be assessed after two weeks, and antibiotic treatment should only be continued in case of a clinical benefit, otherwise the treatment should be stopped. It is important to avoid repeated use of antibiotics such as fluoroquinolones if there is no obvious symptom benefit or other evidence from clinical chemistry or culture tests that supports an infectious etiology.

GP. What is the optimal management of nonbacterial prostatitis patients?

UR. The management of chronic prostatitis/chronic pelvic pain syndrome (CP/CPPS) is indeed challenging. Our understanding of the etiology and pathogene-sis of this condition remains inadequate, and current treatment strategies are fre-quently ineffective. There are a lot of treatment options reported in the recent literature, such as alpha-blockers, antibiotics, phytotherapy, anti-inflammatory drugs, pentosan polysulfate, and others. Some authors have focused on the elimination of specific risk factors that come from the diet and that are related to sexual habits, general lifestyle, and repeated perineal trauma causing pelvic floor muscle tenderness (i.e., bicycling). Some physical treatments, such as extracorporeal shockwave therapy or electroacupuncture or psychological treatment, have also been reported. However, the best results can be obtained by using a clinical phenotype-based classification system including six domains (urinary, psychosocial, organ specific, infection, neurologic/systemic, and tenderness) (UPOINT). Based on this innovative classification system, there is growing evidence for a benefit of an integrated team approach to assess and manage these patients according to their individual symptom pattern or phenotype.

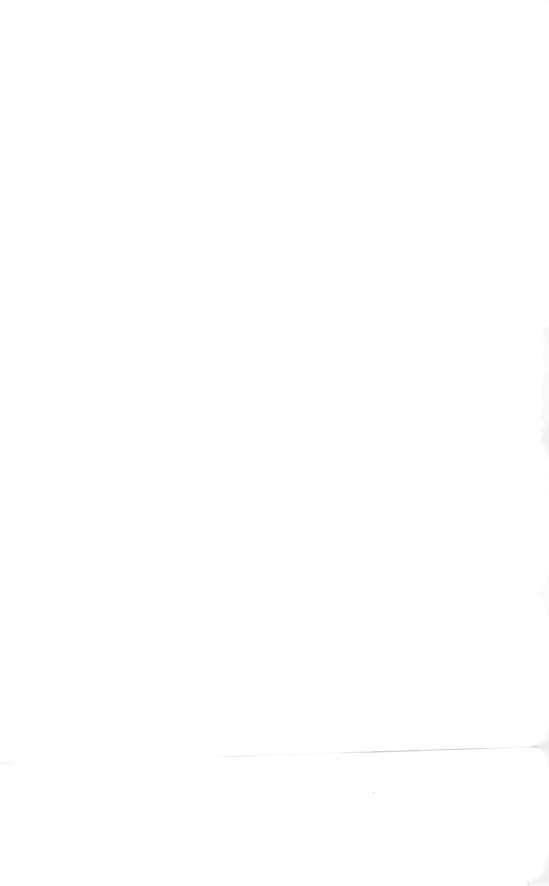

Printed in the United States
By Bookmasters